Backyard Food Security

How to Turn Dead Soil, Tubs, and Lawns into a Personal Food Safety System

Marko Vovk

This publication is intended to provide accurate and authoritative information on the subject matter covered. It is sold with the understanding that the author and publisher are not providing legal or medical advice. Readers should consult qualified professionals regarding their own situations.

For permission requests, visit: clevelanandmold@aol.com

Paperback: ISBN: 978-1-969955-34-1

E-Book: ISBN: 978-1-969955-35-8

Cover design: Marko Vovk (Draft 2, 5-1-26 Chapters 16 and 17 added) Interior design: Marko Vovk. Final editing by Marko Vovk (some minor inconsistencies may remain; no outside paid editor was used). Printed in the United States of America.

Portions of this material are adapted from earlier works by the author, including *Fix Your Toxic Home and Live Longer*, *Poisoned at the Grocery Store*, *Poisoned at the Restaurant*, *Forever Chemicals – How PFAS Pollutes Our Blood and Lives*, *The Water You Drink May Be Killing You*, *Pressure Canning – Safe Preservation of Food at Home*, *No-Mow Living – The Real Hidden Costs of Grass*, and *The Duck Who Watched*, together with insights drawn from more than 18,000 home inspections over the last 45 years.

Contents

Introduction

Why Your Yard Still Matters

In 1943, ordinary people grew almost half of America's vegetables in yards, school lots, and community patches. They did this with shovels, seed, and jars, not apps or plastic clamshells. Today, the same country relies on distant fields, bomb-age fertilizer, trucks, and factories for every bite. We traded rows of beans for rectangles of shaved grass and acted surprised when empty shelves and bad ingredients showed up on the same bill.

This book looks at this trade from both ends. First, it walks through how much homegrown food we lost in one human lifetime. It shows how to build a personal food safety system from the soil up, even if you only have tubs, a small yard, or a balcony. The goal is not a postcard garden or a trendy raised bed full of store-bought mix. The goal is plates of real food you control, grown in soil that heals rather than collapses.

I grew up in the shadow of people who remembered hunger and ration lines. My Slovenian mother sent me out to the yard for lettuce and tomatoes before dinner and stacked jars in the basement like bricks. Later, I watched the world pulled apart by cheap fuel, bright supermarkets, and lawns that never fed anyone.

I spent decades inspecting houses and seeing what lies under the grass: compacted fill, tired soil, and a thin layer of roots trying to make sense of it. Those years taught me one thing. The story of food is always the story of soil and who controls it.

You will not find glossy "perfect garden" pictures in these pages. You will see mounds built on dead corners start working again. You will see chop and drop beds hold water while bare plots bleach and crack. You will meet compost cores and keyhole gardens that turn kitchen scraps and rinse water into steady harvests.

You will see rotation in tubs, simple seed saving, and home food preservation used as tools in a larger system, not as hobbies. Each piece stands on its own, yet they all serve one job: to move power back from factories and boardrooms into your hands and your yard.

The system you live in now runs on a different plan. Fertilizer plants built for war found a new life selling nitrogen, phosphorus, and potash as "plant food." Corporations learned to strip fields, ship crops, process them, and send them back in cans and boxes loaded with salt, sugar, oils, coatings, and stabilizers.

Landscapes filled with lawns that demand fuel, chemicals, and weekend mowing instead of giving you dinner. The results stain rivers, build dead zones offshore, and push nitrate and other pollutants into wells. The same pattern that hurts water and soil also leaves your plate dependent on long chains of people you will never meet.

You cannot fix it on your own. You can change how much it owns you. A small set of simple moves makes a bigger difference than most people want to admit. Cut crops at the base and leave roots in place. Stack lasagna mounds on the worst ground instead of digging deeper.

Sprinkle in a little forest soil and protect the surface with armor. Add a compost heart or wood core where you can, so beds feed themselves. Rotate families through tubs and pools. Save seed from what thrives. Learn enough about canning, freezing, and drying to turn a short harvest into a long eating window. None of this requires a farm. All of it adds weight to your side of the scale.

This is not a book about perfection. My own plots have bad seasons, failed experiments, and weeds that slip in. Some years disease hits hard. Other years time or health falls short. A mound that gave a squash crop one summer might stall a different plant the next. Garlic cloves rot under too much straw. Seedlings fail. That is normal. The point is not to win every season. The point is to move from a flat, fragile setup that fails all at once to a layered system that can take hits and keep feeding you.

You also will not see many fancy gadgets here. Most of what I use comes from municipal leaf piles, old tubs, soft pools, simple mesh, and local seed houses. I want you to see that you can build working soil with what your town throws away and what your own kitchen already produces. You do not need a subscription box, a designer kit, or a new power tool to start. You need a patch of light, some patience, and a willingness to let biology work rather than fight it with steel and salts.

Here is how the book unfolds. The opening chapters show how home gardens once fed America and how bomb plants, chemical fertilizers, and big lawns broke the link. Later chapters move under your feet into the underground city of microbes, fungi, worms, and roots that still run every real harvest.

From there, we climb back to the surface to look at chop and drop armor, healing mounds, wood core variations, and self feeding keyhole designs. We stretch out into companion planting, mixed plots, cover crops, and rotation, scaled down to small beds and containers. The last chapter walks through seed saving and home preservation and ends with a simple question. Do you want the store as your lifeline, or as backup for the edges your yard cannot yet handle?

When you reach the last page, you should be able to look at whatever space you have and see a path forward. Maybe you live on a city lot with tired clay and strict rules. Maybe you have a strip of ground, a few soft pools on gravel, or three windows that catch decent sun. Maybe you already grow and can but want a system that wastes less water and holds up better in hard years. Wherever you start, the steps in this book can help you build a personal food safety system, one bed, one jar, and one habit at a time.

You do not have to quit stores or raise all your calories. You do not have to copy every pattern or every number. Take what matches your climate, body, and time. Test it on a small scale. Keep what works, and move on from what does not. That is how real soil, real gardens, and real independence grow. The next chapter begins where this whole story went off track: the years when ordinary people turned lawns into food, and how fast that power was given away.

Chapter 1: When Gardens Fed America

How Families Turned Lawns into Food

In 1943, home gardens grew about 42 percent of the vegetables eaten in the United States. The country held 133 million people, not today's swollen count. About 21 million Victory Gardens covered 8 million acres and raised close to 10 billion pounds of vegetables in one focused season. Almost half the nation's vegetables came from yards, school lots, and community patches instead of trucks and factories.

Many of those gardeners were recent or first generation immigrants who had walked through Ellis Island a few decades earlier. They came from farm families in Europe and elsewhere and brought hard lessons in their bones. They had smelled real hunger and watched ration lines snake around blocks. Two world wars and food shortages had taught them what empty shelves meant. When officials called for

Victory Gardens, these families did not need glossy flyers to explain why.

The Roosevelt administration turned gardening into blunt wartime policy. Federal agencies blasted messages on posters, radio, and in pamphlets. Lawns, vacant lots, and rooftops were targets, not decorations. The pitch stayed simple and harsh. Grow food here so more canned meat, grain, and oil can go to soldiers and allies overseas. Do your duty with a shovel, or watch someone else's child go hungry.

I came along later as a baby boomer, born after that wave of urgency. In the 1960s, many homes on my street still lined their backs with rows instead of play sets. My Slovenian mother had grown up on a farm and never trusted a store as much as she trusted her own hands. Before many dinners, she sent me out to the yard to grab lettuce, tomatoes, or peppers. Salad did not mean a plastic box. It meant whatever I could carry in from the damp soil behind the garage.

Canning rose with those rows. In 1943 alone, families and community centers filled more than 4.1 billion jars. Early in the war, pressure canners were scarce. Near the end, factories turned out hundreds of thousands, and mason jars were stacked like bricks on basement shelves. A single block of small houses in a city might hold tens of thousands of sealed jars. Each one meant a little less power for ration cards, bottling plants, and middlemen.

Then the knives came out for that culture. Through the 1950s and 1960s, home gardens started to shrink and then vanish. More women took jobs outside the home and had fewer hours to weed, cook from scratch, and stand over boiling kettles. New supermarkets promised bright aisles of cheap, endless food.

You could trade a weekend in the yard for a fluorescent cart and a frozen dinner. Television ads painted jars and dirt as backward, while frozen pies and boxed mixes stood for success. Big agriculture stepped forward with larger fields, more chemicals, and the promise that faraway farms and factories could feed every table. Lawns and ornamental shrubs rolled over beans and cabbage like carpet bombing.

The population changed at the same time. The country did not pass 300 million people until long after the war years. Baby boomers filled the gap between 133 million and today's 330 plus million. Most of that crowd grew up closer to grocery coolers than to grandparents' fields. Garden skills stayed within a few stubborn families but bled out of school lessons, magazines, and television. Food became something wrapped, branded, and scanned instead of picked, washed, and jarred.

Today, the United States has a population of about 335 million people. The canning jar business pulls in around 1 billion dollars per year and may climb toward 1.5 billion, but that shine hides a hollow center. Fewer than half of households put away anything in a year, and many of those fill only a few jars for fun rather than for real storage.

Home plots now grow only a thin single digit share of the nation's vegetables, down from that old 42 percent. In less than a century, 30 points of production slid from backyards into distant industrial fields and processing plants. Control followed the crops.

The reasons run deeper than laziness. Cheap fuel made it possible to drag produce thousands of miles and still undercut local efforts. Chemical fertilizers and pesticides let exhausted fields limp along long enough to keep store shelves full.

Food companies learned to add salt, sugar, oils, and stabilizers to products so they could sit for months and still look fresh. Whole generations learned to trust labels more than their grandparents did. The system taught people that real dirt was optional and that real cooking belonged on old black and white shows.

In 1943, ordinary people used shovels and jars to flood their own plates with food. Today, most of that power sits in factories, trucks, and boardrooms. The next chapter steps into the engine room of that shift. It shows how bomb plants and fertilizer bags turned soil from partner to patient and hooked both farmers and eaters on a steady drip of chemicals.

Chapter 2: Bomb Plants and Fertilizer Bags

How Explosives Became Plant Food

Chapter 2: Bomb Plants and Fertilizer Bags
Subheading: How Explosives Became Plant Food

World War II left behind vast nitrate and ammonia factories built to load shells and bombs, not to grow dinner. When the shooting stopped, those nitrogen rivers did not dry up. They changed labels. Plants that had churned out explosives for artillery and aerial bombs were now rebranded as "plant food" and pushed into the soil instead of steel. Big operations leaned hard on these salts each season, chasing bigger harvests for a swelling nation.

The new chemistry looked clean on paper. Ammonium nitrate and anhydrous ammonia delivered fast nitrogen hits once used to blow holes in cities and bunkers. Urea offered dense nitrogen that spread. Superphosphate and its triple strength cousin brought concentrated phosphorus. Muriate and sulfate of potash supplied potassium in tight grains. Corn, wheat, and soy absorbed these inputs as cities filled with baby boom mouths. The sales pitch sounded irresistible. Add more product, pull more grain, feed the empire.

Stories dressed this shift up as destiny, not as a choice. Government experts praised "scientific farming" in glossy pamphlets. Company ads promised "bumper crops with less work" and "modern plant food for modern farms." Suburban pitches dangled "golf course lawns" and "lush green in days." Fertility in a sack. Food and status on demand. The quiet message under every slogan stayed the same. Old ways were backward. Real progress came in bright printed packages.

Those sacks stepped off fields and onto every cul de sac. Farm blends found their way into hardware stores and new garden centers. Shelves groaned under weed and feed, starter lawn formulas, and "all purpose" mixes. Cartoon vegetables and grinning turf smiled from the front. Families traded mixed rows of beans, onions, and cabbage for smooth rectangles of shaved grass. Saturday morning turned into mower time, not planting time. I later wrote Grass Be Gone and No Mow Living after watching bright turf roll over soil and food, but here the question cuts deeper. What did those perfect green carpets do to land, water, and bodies?

This chemistry does not stop at a property line. Crops take up only part of the nitrogen they receive. Much of the rest rides off in rain and snowmelt, through ditches and streams, and into major rivers. That flow now helps drive a Gulf of Mexico "dead zone" that can cover 5,000 to 8,000 square miles most summers. Some years, the oxygen starved patch reaches the size of a small state. Fish flee if they can outrun it. Bottom life suffocates in place.

The leaks show up inland too. Runoff from fields and chemically treated grass now feeds slime green blooms in lakes across the Midwest and beyond. Brown tap water warnings flash in towns that never saw such colors before. Nitrate from fertilizer and manure seeps into aquifers and private wells. Millions of Americans drink water contaminated with elevated nitrate levels, even if they never load a spreader in their yard. Health agencies link exposure to blue baby syndrome, certain cancers, thyroid problems, and gut stress in children and pregnant women. Some communities near major ammonia and nitrate plants now report higher than average cancer and respiratory illness rates, stacking factory air atop polluted water.

A few names sit at the center of this river. Nutrien sells fertilizer across continents and controls large chunks of potash and retail sales in North America. Mosaic mines and markets a major slice of phosphorus and potash for broad acre operations. CF Industries ships huge volumes of ammonia and urea to growers who often see no realistic alternative. Yara is a nitrogen giant that sells "nutrition solutions" to more than 20 million clients worldwide. A tight cluster of corporations handles a large part of the global nutrient valve and profits every time someone feels they cannot grow food without another application.

As a Boy Scout in the 1960s, I helped carry this new normal door to door. Our troop raised money by selling lawn formulas and weed killers in tidy bags. We knocked, smiled, and walked away as garages filled with more jugs and sacks. No one talked about stream health, well tests, or soil biology at those meetings. We measured success in total pounds moved. At home, my mother still trusted compost piles, kitchen scraps, and careful watering. One yard ran on stories and seeds. Many others ran on slogans and sprays.

Explosives turned into everyday "plant food" in less than a generation. Shaved grass replaced kitchen rows. Runoff carried stray nitrogen and phosphorus toward rivers, wells, and seabed's. A small circle of companies learned how to sell dependence by the ton and call it progress. The next chapter moves under that bright surface, into the dark networks of fungi and microbes that once fed Victory Gardens without any chemical help at all.

Chapter 3: The Underground City

Fungi, Microbes, and the Hidden Engine

Press your thumb into damp earth, and you touch a city. One teaspoon can hold about 1 billion bacteria and up to 50,000 kinds of microbes. Names like Bacillus, Pseudomonas, and Rhizobium work beside countless nameless cousins. This city never sleeps. It hums under every step, even when the top looks like dead dust.

Down in that layer, each crew has a role. Bacteria and fungi break down old roots and fallen leaves, turning them into usable nutrients. Protozoa and small worms graze on those microbes and release pulses of plant food beside the finest root hairs. Sticky films from bacterial and fungal webs glue particles into crumbs that catch air and trap water. Tiny insects and other arthropods shred debris and carve tunnels where air and new roots can move. Together, they turn loose dust into a stable, breathing skeleton that supports life.

"Mycorrhizal" sounds like lab talk, but it means one thing. Fungus root. These partners wrap themselves around and into root systems and sign a trade deal. The host sends sugars made from sunlight. In return, the fungi build long, fine networks called hyphae that stretch far past the root tips. Each strand is thinner than a hair yet can run for feet through narrow pores.

Those networks act like a second root system that the plant never had to grow. Trials show mycorrhizal fungi can double phosphorus uptake when the ground runs short. Growth can jump by about 50 percent when roots are well colonized. The fungal web also carries warning signals and carbon between neighbors, linking separate stems into a quiet underground internet. It behaves like a living pipeline, not a passive sponge.

Bomb age salts smashed into this web in ways bag labels never mentioned. High phosphorus fertilizer can reduce mycorrhizal colonization by 30 percent or more. Heavy nitrogen doses shorten hyphae and blunt their reach through the ground. Deep tillage and bare patches rip fungal routes apart and speed the burn off of stored carbon. You get quick green on top, but weak support below. The city still stands, yet whole neighborhoods go dark.

Forest inoculation shows how little it can take to steer this system back. In one trial, researchers spread less than 1 centimeter of healthy donor soil over damaged land. Within about six years, plant communities shifted toward the original grassland or heath. The mix of bacteria, fungi, and worms changed too, not just the stems and leaves above. A thin dusting of living material turned a wrecked field back toward its old self.

You can run a small version at home. Walk into a strong woodland and look for deep leaf layers and dark, rich earth. Scoop a trowel or two of that material and bring it back. Sprinkle it over your bed, then cover it with mulch to keep it moist and shaded. You seed your yard with a starter culture, the way a spoonful of yogurt seeds a fresh batch of milk. That forest city starts to throw branches across your raised beds and pots.

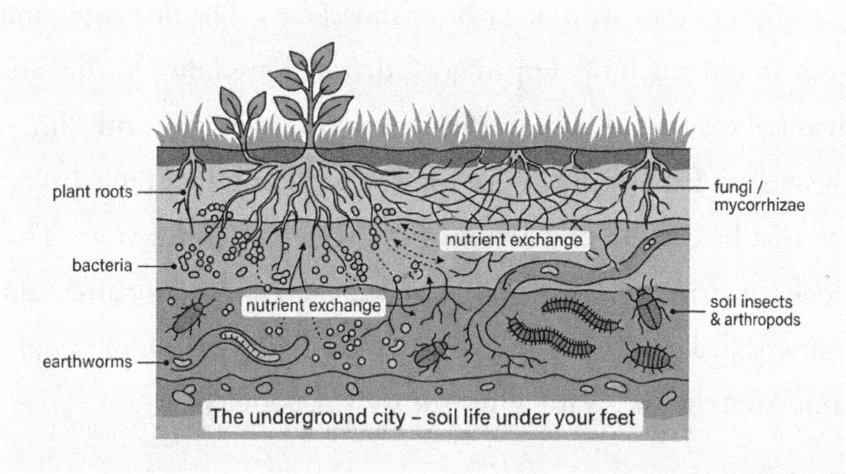

My own growing space runs on that idea. I skip chemical fertilizers. I use leaf humus that has aged for one to two years in large municipal piles. A nearby city vacuums leaves from curbs, turns them, and gives the finished material away. Each year, my ground level sinks a little as life eats and shrinks the old organic matter. Each year, I haul in a pickup load of dark, crumbling humus and spread it over my big beds. The response shows up in thick root systems, strong color, and steady yields without bright bags. Smaller plots can do the same with a wheelbarrow pulled from a forest edge or a local leaf pile.

The payoff goes far beyond a nice look. A biologically active acre can carry tons of microscopic life, equal to or more than a herd of livestock underfoot. Mycorrhizal networks and bacterial crews release phosphorus and nitrogen that already sit locked in the mineral bank. Stable crumbs hold more water and air, so roots neither drown nor dry out as quickly. With a strong underground city, crops need less extra fertilizer and less constant irrigation to stay upright.

I saw the contrast with one pair of shovel cuts. The first slice came from an old patch of clipped grass that had lived on mowing and chemical treatments. The profile looked pale and tight, with almost no smell and almost no visible roots. The second slice came from a bed that had taken leaves, humus, and gentle tools for years. That block fell apart in dark crumbs, smelled like a forest floor after rain, and wriggled with small worms when light struck it. Both samples came from the same yard. Only the treatment differed.

The bomb age trained people to pour nutrients from above and ignore the life below. This buried city points to another route. Seed the community, protect it, and let it rebuild its own networks and banks. The next chapter moves from invisible webs to one straightforward move you can start today. Cut crops at the base, leave them as armor, and feed this underground city instead of stripping its food away.

Chapter 4: Chop and Drop Armor

How Leaving Plants Saves Soil

One of the simplest tricks costs nothing and scares fertilizer companies. Every dead crop can become protection and food for the bed. A blanket of chopped plant matter on top can reduce water loss to about 40 percent of bare ground in the first days after watering. That same cover can slash erosion by more than three quarters during hard rain.

Chop and drop means crops stop going in the trash can. When a row finishes, cut the stems at the base and leave the roots in place to hold the ground. Chop stalks and leaves into smaller pieces. Drop that cut up mass right where it grew as a loose blanket. No plastic bags. No hauling. No naked ground. The floor starts to look more like a forest, where nothing leaves and nothing stays exposed.

Trials with different coverings give numbers to this lazy method. In container tests, a layer about 5 centimeters deep cut evaporation from the top to 40 percent of the loss from uncovered mix during the first few days. Field studies found that protected plots lost 75 to 98 percent less soil than bare test strips during intense storms or on new slopes. Unprotected ground bled tons of sediment per hectare, while mulched patches hardly moved. The difference did not come from a magic product. It came from refusing to strip away what the crop had already grown.

In my own beds, nothing green leaves the system, even in large containers. Twenty forty gallon above ground pots line my rows, small enough for one person to tip when empty. Weeds and soft trimmings go into the bottom of those tubs, not into trash sacks. Fresh plant scraps go in first, then I pour last year's used potting mix from another container over them. By the next year, when I empty or flip that tub, the buried layer has turned into dark, crumbly earth ready for another round. Most growers use fixed beds they cannot move, so they rebuild in place. Portable pots let me stack the process, but the rule stays the same. Keep organic matter close and working.

Another engine runs behind this. A nearby farm piles horse manure year after year. The oldest front edge, four to five years old, stays packed with earthworms. A small shovelful of that aged, worm rich material goes into each pot before planting a new crop. Those worms handle daily tillage without steel. They drag fragments downward, mix layers, and leave castings that hold water and nutrients better than the original blend.

Some containers need extra protection over winter. In the fall, I cover garlic tubs with a layer of straw to shield cloves from harsh cold. The straw brings a few hitchhiking seeds, so grass blades pop up in spring. I pull those invaders as soon as they threaten herbs or vegetables and throw them back on top to dry. Sun kills the roots, and the remains melt into future soil. In other years, fallen leaves took the place of straw, but I do not have big trees. Fresh leaves arrive only when I rescue bagged piles from other yards.

Under all that cover, the buried city from the last chapter keeps getting fed. Microbes colonize chopped stems and start breaking them down. Worms pull small bits into their burrows and leave castings rich in nutrients and firm crumbs. Over time, this slow rain of organic matter builds structure, boosts water holding, and smooths temperature swings at the surface. Weeds also lose ground. A few centimeters of mixed cover can block much of the light that weed seeds need to sprout.

Many growers fear that leaving dead growth will invite disease and pests. A soaked, matted layer pressed tight against stems can cause trouble. A dry, loose blanket often does the opposite. It blocks muddy splash, one of the main routes leaf diseases use to reach new growth. Many insects that chew leaves hate the cooler, shaded conditions under cover and move on. Slugs and rodents can build up in thick, wet mats, so watch for that and thin the blanket or switch to a different material if needed.

When there is more chopped plant material than a bed can handle, you do not stuff it deeper. Extra goes to a compost heap, where it breaks down into finished humus for later use. Chop and drop turns every crop into a tool that keeps working after harvest. Stalks become shade, leaves become armor, and roots become future tunnels.

The underground city receives steady food, and the surface stops bleeding water and soil. The next chapter shows how to combine this armor with a small dose of forest earth so each bed not only keeps its skin but also inherits a living starter culture from one of nature's best teachers.

Chapter 5: Healing Mound Gardens

Growing Food Without Breaking Soil

Some ground never seems to forgive. You loosen it, dress it, water it, and it still crusts, puddles, and strangles roots. Old lawn, compacted fill, and cheap trucked "topsoil" can all act this way. The issue is not only lack of nutrients. The earth's body is damaged. Digging deeper with blades and machines does not cure that. Building upward lets the land repair itself from below.

Deep tilling behaves more like mining than care. Each pass shatters natural layers that once kept water and air in balance. Buried organic matter comes into contact with oxygen and burns off as gas. Dark crumbs smear into dust that wind and storm steal. In many long worked fields, the rich band has thinned or vanished. Every heavy tilling makes the soil looser for one season and poorer for the next. Small yards repeat the same mistake with a rototiller every spring.

Mounds offer a way out without endless truckloads. A curved surface warms faster in spring than a flat one because more of it catches the sun. Cold, wet patches can stay stubborn while the dome dries and warms enough to take seed. Water shifts, too. It slides off the curve and sinks near the base instead of pooling in the middle. That helps on tight or compacted sites where rain often sits and suffocates roots. Inside, roots can dive into the old hard layer and explore sideways into the softer fill stacked on top.

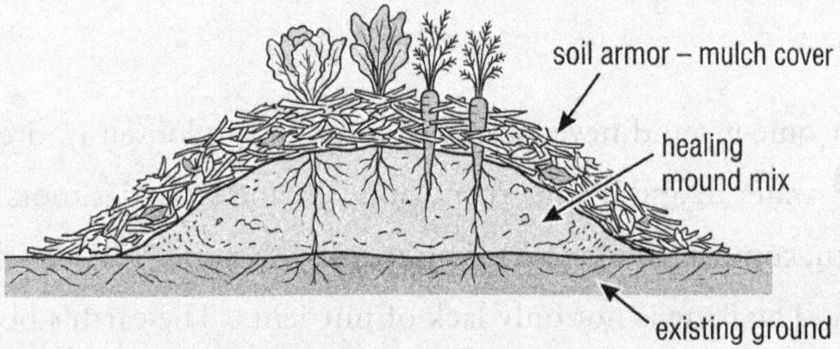

Healing mound with soil armor – side view.

Building a no till mound over bad ground is like stacking a lasagna. Mark a circle or oval on the stubborn patch. If tough grass or weeds dominate, lay down one sheet of cardboard or heavy paper to slow them, but do not smother the area. On that mark, pile a loose mat of rough organic scraps: small sticks, dry stalks, sunflower stems, pruned twigs. This base creates pockets and slow rot, not instant compost. Above that, add richer material such as compost, aged manure, leaf humus, or used potting mix that still has some life. Shape a low dome about 20 to 30 centimeters high, with gentle slopes, and firm it lightly so it holds its form while still breathing.

Some growers push this further by tucking old wood inside. Partially rotted logs and thick branches act like nurse logs in a forest. As they break down, they absorb water like a sponge and slowly release it back into the mound. Trials on buried wood systems show decomposed softwood can hold several times its dry weight in water, keeping the surrounding mix moist long after plain earth in the same weather dries out. In a dry spell, that buried sponge can mean the difference between wilted plants and steady growth.

The move is simple. On a site with clean, untreated wood, lay a few short pieces across the base layer of sticks before adding richer material. Skip black walnut, pressure treated boards, painted scraps, or lumber of unknown history. Cover the wood completely so it never sees light. Over the years, fungi and microbes eat into the grain, turning it into a soft, dark mass that stores moisture and feeds the mound from within. Roots thread through those pockets, exploring old root channels.

In my above ground pools and large tubs, I do not have room for big logs, but I use the same idea in smaller form. A layer of coarse wood chips at the bottom of deep containers holds extra moisture and slowly breaks down into rich material. It does not store as much water as a full log, yet it still turns dead space into a reservoir and food bank. If you have more room in a fixed bed, you can move from chips to short branch sections buried low in the mound and let time do the rest. Your plot becomes one more experiment that shows how much wood your mix will welcome.

The dome is still a shell until it gets a living pattern. Forest starter soil brings that pattern in. Do not raid parks or fragile preserves. Go to ordinary woods, hedgerows, or shelterbelts with deep leaf carpets. Lift the leaf layer and skim a very thin slice of dark earth from several spots. Avoid taking big shovels from one place. Back at the mound, crumble those handfuls across the top in a light scatter, just enough to speckle the surface. Cover with a loose dressing of dry plant matter such as straw, shredded stems, or chopped leaves. That dusting of wild soil carries a blueprint for structure and life.

Planting can welcome or choke this design. Give roots reasons to meet by spacing crops so their underground zones overlap. Tall species like corn or sunflowers can sit near the center, with beans or other climbers at their feet and lower growers such as squash or herbs along the shoulders. Long season crops do better in these mounds than very quick ones because fungal partners and other allies need time to run through the new space. Skip high phosphorus starter blends. If crops ask for help, lay on gentle additions to the surface, such as compost or light doses of low salt liquid feed. Keep metal and shovels shallow. Open narrow holes for transplants or stakes, but do not drive tools deep through the heart.

Over time, you can see whether a mound has begun to heal the ground under it. After a pounding storm, water will slide off the sides, but the earth at the base should stay in place rather than wash into streaks. Slide a trowel in near the edge. The old hard layer should give way more easily than when you began. During dry spells, cracks that once split the surface may shrink or disappear because the dome and the zone below hold moisture better. New life often shows up. Mushrooms or fine fungal threads may appear at the edges. Volunteer seedlings you never planted can sprout near the base, drawn by better conditions. Those signs mean you built more than a pile. You built a scaffold for recovery.

I tested this in a corner that defeated every crop. The fill there came from a cheap truckload spread after work near the house. It looked dark for a year and then settled into something like hardened cake. Peppers, beans, and cabbage would sprout and then stall halfway to full size. I stopped attacking it with tools and stacked a mound on top. Rough stalks went down first, then compost and old potting mix. I dusted the top with small handfuls of woodland soil and mulched. Squash and a few beans went in, and I left the dome alone except for water and light feeding from above.

In the first season, the mound held moisture better, and the squash reached harvest. In the second year, a test cut with the trowel showed that the old layer beneath had softened, and roots had run deeper. A third season brought fewer puddles, less cracking around the mound, and plants did not stall halfway through summer. That corner stepped back from dead zone to working ground without one more pass of the tiller.

Self healing structures need steady care, not constant reinvention. Each year, after harvest, add a thin layer of organic matter: spent vines, shredded stems, or compost. Cut crops at the base and leave their roots in place to rot into new channels. When the dome settles low after several seasons, top it up with more rough fill and richer material, and let the pattern drive deeper into the old layer. Deep digging does not return to these spots. Treat them as long term projects that gain value with age, like seasoned cast iron or well kept tools.

Beds that repair themselves do more than grow food. They undo some of the damage caused by compaction and careless mixing. They shelter roots, help water soak in, and host unseen allies that extend every plant's reach. Once a few of these mounds are working, you can fill them with partners who take on a second job for you. The next chapter shifts above ground to those allies, the flowers and herbs that stand guard against insects so you spray less and harvest more.

Chapter 6: Companion Pest Shields

Let Plants Do the Bug Work

Some beds feel cursed. Aphids coat tender tips. Hornworms strip leaves in one night. You knock them back, they return. Change the cast, and the story changes. Flowers, herbs, and strong scented crops can confuse pests, feed their enemies, and pull more pollinators into your space. A smart mix turns one row into a quiet defense system that works while you sleep.

Insects do not wander. Many follow smell and leaf chemistry to find food. Strong herbs like basil, rosemary, and sage send out competing signals, making it harder for pests to latch onto a single host. Umbel flowers and small composite blooms drip nectar and pollen for hunters and "bodyguards" such as parasitic wasps, hoverflies, and lady beetles. These allies need sugar and protein to fuel patrols. Strips of blossoms and herb clumps act as service stations where they refuel between hunts. Bees and butterflies also crowd into those same patches, so each guard post doubles as a pollinator magnet.

Some partnerships have moved from folklore into trials. Basil grown with tomatoes has boosted growth, stiffened stems, and improved root systems in several tests while also cutting chewing damage. Marigolds, especially certain French types, can suppress root knot nematodes when grown as a solid stand or in rotation. Yields in some crops jumped by up to half when marigolds preceded or shared space with vulnerable species. Onions, chives, and garlic emit strong odors that repel or confuse aphids and whiteflies near tomatoes and peppers. These combinations do not erect invisible walls. They make it harder for pests to follow the path to your food.

Trap crops work the opposite angle. Instead of pushing attackers away, they lure them to the wrong table. Nasturtiums draw aphids, flea beetles, and some caterpillars far more eagerly than many vegetables. Planted along edges or in sacrificial patches, they act as decoys. You check those first. When they load up, you prune, crush, or haul out the worst sections or even remove the whole clump. That keeps outbreaks tight and visible, instead of letting them creep across your main crop.

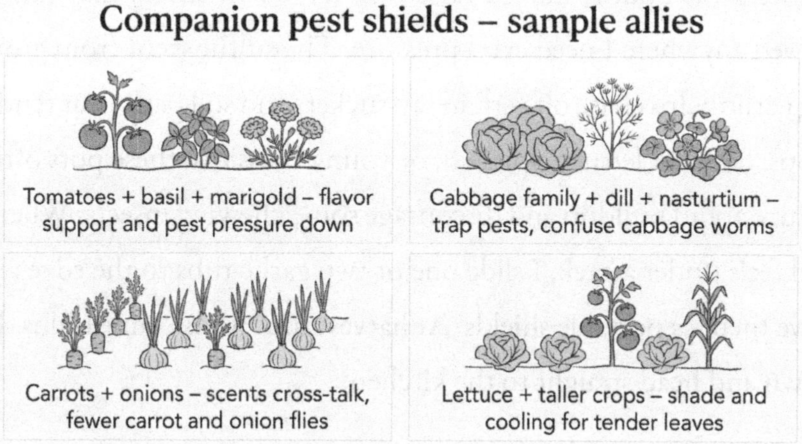

Border flowers do more than decorate. Dill, fennel, cilantro, yarrow, alyssum, and cosmos offer nectar and pollen on open, easy access heads. Tiny wasps that lay eggs in caterpillars need those resources between attacks. Hoverflies, whose larvae can strip aphid colonies, rely on nectar as adults. When these patches bloom near your vegetables, predators linger longer. They do not have to fly far for fuel between pest patrols. Pollinators also key in on these borders, which can lift fruit set on crops that need visits to fill pods, ears, or fruit.

In my beds, these allies do more than guard. They also stock the pantry. Through the warm months, I grow big blocks of basil, mint, lemon balm, and other herbs. Later, I dry and grind them into winter teas and kitchen mixes. Marigold petals are added to some of those blends and salves. The same green guardians steady the insect world in summer and extend their value deep into winter. Their work starts as defense and ends as medicine and flavor.

Garlic pulls double duty. I raise it in large containers that can be moved anywhere I need extra pressure. The sulfur scent from growing garlic helps chase off certain sap suckers and soil pests near tender crops. Set near lettuce, spinach, or young brassicas, these pots often reduce aphid buildup and discourage some chewing insects. When a bed feels under attack, I slide one or two garlic tubs to the edge and leave them as portable shields. At harvest time, those same bulbs dry down and head straight to the kitchen.

Some of my favorite mixed defenses live in soft pools. These fabric circles hold about 100 gallons of growing mix, stand 35 centimeters tall, and span about 1.5 meters across. In one, I often plant onions over part of the surface and leafy crops like lettuce or herbs over the rest. Marigolds or other bloomers anchor the rim. The onions bring scent and shallow feeding. Leafy greens cover the surface and shade the ground. The flowers pull in pollinators and insect allies. That one pool becomes a dense neighborhood where every stem has a job.

Not every famous pairing earns its legend. Some claims rest solely on tradition and fall apart when results are measured. Mixed planting does not make crops untouchable. It tilts the odds. Beds that layer scents, nectar stations, traps, and strong root smells tend to slow outbreaks and reduce the frequency of interventions. Your job is to test combinations in small patches, keep notes, and expand what works in your climate and soil while ignoring the myths that fall flat.

One season showed how this shift plays out. The first year, a long tomato row stood somewhat naked, with bare ground below and only stakes beside it. Hornworms and aphids hit hard. I picked, sprayed organic soaps, and still lost foliage. The next year, I broke that row into sections. Basil went to the feet of many tomatoes. Marigolds slipped between every few plants. Dill and onions lined the edge, with a strip of nasturtiums as bait. Hornworms appeared, but fewer and later. Aphids landed, but hoverfly larvae and tiny wasps held their numbers down. My hands still mattered, yet the spray bottle stayed on the shelf. The plants and their allies took most of the load.

Companion pest shields do not replace vigilance. They change the battlefield in your favor. You stack scents and blooms, set decoys, and feed the hunters so they stay on patrol. Once beds carry these living shields, you can push the idea further. The next chapter scales that thinking to whole patches where multiple crops share ground in ways that feed people, protect soil, and cut nutrient loss in one pattern.

Chapter 7: Three Sisters Power Plots

Corn, Beans, and Squash on One Patch

Walk any grocery aisle, and you see corn, beans, and squash stacked in bright steel. The labels look harmless. The contents often do not. Many brands drag in field pesticides, can coatings, excess salt, sugar, gums, and other stabilizers. Some use patented, genetically engineered crop lines designed for machines, not for human health.

I dug into these hidden layers in my book, *Poisoned at the Grocery Store: What They Added and Never Told You*, which tracks how food changes from field to cart. The more you learn about those additions, the more sense it makes to grow these staples in your own ground with no invisible extras riding along.

Three Sisters planting is not a random tangle. Indigenous growers across North America refined this trio over generations. Corn stands upright and forms the scaffold. Climbing beans wind around the stalks, add protein to the harvest, and host nitrogen fixing bacteria on their roots. Squash sprawls across the ground, shades the surface, holds moisture, and slows weed growth. Corn brings energy. Beans bring protein. Squash provides vitamins, fiber, and oil rich seeds. Together, they build whole meals that can carry through winter in a cellar or pantry without dyes, coatings, or preservatives.

Seed choice sits at the center of this pattern. Heirloom and other open pollinated lines make seed that grows like the parent as long as you keep crosses under control. When you save from the best hills and replant, the next crop stays true in shape, flavor, and timing. Over the years, those lines bend toward your exact soil and weather. Hybrids play a different game. They come from a carefully constructed line bred for one season of performance. The children split. Hybrid seed saved often produces uneven, weak, or off type plants. Some barely produce. Many modern commercial offerings are hybrids or protected types. That keeps you buying each year instead of building your own family.

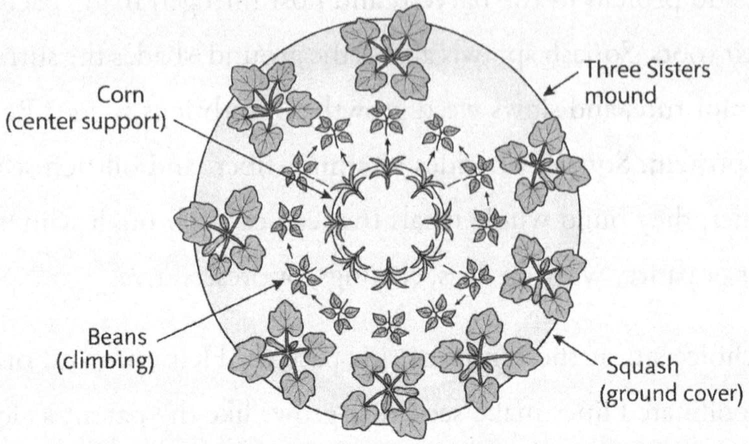

In a Three Sisters plot, open pollinated, untreated, non GMO seed matters. It lets you carry corn, beans, and squash seed forward and step away from yearly dependence on catalogs.

Corn in this pattern has to act as both grain and stake. Modern sweet types bred for supermarket ears often grow tall and soft, snapping under the weight of beans or a gusty storm. Older flour and flint lines bring thicker stalks and better keeping quality. Flour corn dries into tiny kernels that are ground into fine meal for tortillas, pancakes, and baking. Flint types dry hard and glassy, crack into coarse meal or hominy, and hold shape in soups and stews. Many older Indigenous lines sit between those extremes and still give sturdy stalks and good flavor. For this trio, medium height and strong stems matter more than record ear size. The stalk has to carry beans all season without folding.

The bean sister must climb and keep well. Bush types do not fit here. You need vines that can reach up and hold on. Dry pole beans give jars of hard seed that store through winter. Old lines of kidney, pinto, and runners were often chosen with support crops in mind. Their roots form nodules where bacteria capture nitrogen from the air and release some of it into the surrounding soil as roots shed and hosts cycle. That slow trickle can help both corn and squash over a long season. A good Three Sisters bean climbs fast, sets heavy pods, and dries seed before frost in your climate.

Squash in this pattern must cover ground and cure well. The job belongs to rambling winter squash and pumpkins, not compact bush types or soft summer varieties. Vines crawl between hills and weave a living mat over bare earth. Big leaves block light from weed seeds and keep the surface cooler. That canopy holds moisture longer between storms and softens sudden temperature swings. Hard rind winter squash stores for months and is rich in carotene, minerals, and fiber. Their seed offers dense oils and protein. Some older lines were chosen because they spread well between corn clusters without climbing the stalks and dragging them down. Here you want vines roaming over the soil, not up the stems.

The layout decides whether this mix feeds you or fights you. A classic backyard setup uses low mounds. Each dome rises about 30 centimeters above the original grade and spans 45 to 90 centimeters across. The centers are about 1.2 meters apart, so one corn clump does not steal all the light from the next. Corn goes in first, in a small circle near the top. When the young stalks reach about 15 centimeters, the bean seeds form a ring around them. After the squash seeds germinate near the shoulders, the vines can run across the gaps between hills. That spacing gives sun to all three while keeping roots close enough to help each other.

Small spaces force harder choices. Tight beds full of corn and sunflowers can cast such deep shade that nearby crops never reach their potential. That is one reason I do not grow corn or sunflowers in my own garden. My rows and pools are packed with shorter vegetables and herbs that need light all season. Tall stalks would block light, forcing too many trade offs. Some of my colleagues have more room to give this trio the space it needs. They have tested and tuned mounds, distances, and varieties in real earth for years. Their results, along with the long Indigenous record and modern yield studies, make a strong case for including this pattern in a book on soil and independence, even though I have not run a full Three Sisters plot myself.

Canned corn, beans, and squash represent a chain of control you do not own. Crops may come from fields sprayed on tight schedules. Kernels and cubes travel to factories where they meet brine, stabilizers, and lining chemicals. Some cans still raise concerns over compounds that can leach into food. Each step adds risk and cost. In contrast, a small patch of this trio uses heirloom seed, sun, rain, and your labor. You decide what touches the ground and the plants. You decide how clean the irrigation water is, what mulch you drop, and which insects you tolerate. The food on your plate speaks straight from your yard, not from a supply chain scattered across states and countries.

Starting this pattern does not require a field. One or two mounds, a sturdy flour or flint corn, a proven climbing bean, and a vining winter squash are enough to test the idea. Watch where their shade falls, how wind threads through the planting, and how easy it is to reach in for weeding and harvest. Note which stalks handle the bean load and which vines stay on the ground instead of climbing. At the end of the season, choose the best ears, pods, and fruits and keep those seeds for next year. The patch becomes your line, not just a copy of someone else's story.

These power plots ask you to trade neat single rows for a knot of cooperation. In return, you get food, seed control, and a pattern that has proven itself through war, drought, and hunger. The next chapter carries this idea of constant support forward, shifting from mixed crops to year round soil armor so your beds never sit naked waiting for the next hit of stress.

Chapter 8: Soil Armor and Rotational Pots

Cover Crops, Mulch, and Moving Roots in Any Size Garden

Most farms already know one rule. Bare ground means trouble. Many operations now sow cover crops between money makers so the earth does not sit exposed to sun, wind, and pounding rain. They lean on living roots and leftover stalks to build what soil scientists call armor, a shield that keeps the upper band alive and stable. The same idea works on the smallest raised bed or balcony. This kind of protection and rotation is not a farm toy. It is a survival habit for any growing space that wants to keep producing under strange weather and damaged ground.

Real armor means something always guards the bed's skin. On big acreage, that often means a cover crop whose main job is to protect and feed the earth, not fill plates. In a small garden, protection can come from low covers, chopped stalks, and quick swaps that keep root systems on the move. When ground sits naked, every storm, heat wave, and gust steals a little more. With protection in place, energy from sun and rain gets buffered and slowed. Crusting eases, temperature swings soften, and the upper few inches turn crumbly instead of hard. That sponge holds water between storms and lets roots breathe after a downpour.

Most cover stands look modest at first glance. Rye and oats send up narrow blades and tall spires. Clover and vetch creep low and knit a green rug. Buckwheat races ahead with soft stems and white blossoms. None of these land on magazine covers as showcase vegetables. Together, they act like a shield. Foliage intercepts raindrops that would pound bare earth into a sealed crust. Roots tie particles together and push into deeper pockets of water and nutrients. When the stand dies, stalks and buried growth become food for worms and microbes that glue crumbs into sturdy clusters. Each cycle nudges the ground closer to that deep, dark sponge old farmers brag about.

The real engine runs below your boots. Active roots leak sugars as they grow. Those sweet exudates feed bacteria and fungi along the finest hairs. In return, microbes trade nutrients back in a quiet black market under your feet. The more months each year those exchanges run, the steadier the support for crops. Covers stretch that window. They fill gaps between cash rows, between spring harvest and fall sowing, between pulled plants and your next planting date. Instead of feast and famine for underground life, you move toward a steady diet. That steady feed means more toughness when drought hits or when a crop runs into stress.

This chapter leans toward larger gardens and small farms where there is enough space to sow whole strips. Those sites can hold a stand of rye after corn or oats and peas after early potatoes. They can carry clover beneath taller crops and let it regrow once the main harvest is over. The same mindset still serves small backyards, narrow frames, and tubs. A box on legs can wear a thin mat of chopped stalks or a low clover sowing just as a broad field can. The aim is not to mimic big machinery. The aim is to copy the habit. Do not leave the ground naked if you can quickly lay life or residue back on top.

My own layout does not resemble a row crop farm. I run what I call rotational above grade gardens. Instead of long furrows, I use many pots, fabric tubs, and five foot pools packed with a mix of plants. About 1,200 garlic bulbs go into about a third of those containers each year. After planting, I smother those tubs with leaves, straw, or chopped stalks, laid thick enough to hide the soil. That shield keeps winter frost and dry winds from chewing the surface and stops spring storms from splashing material out. When summer heat arrives, the same blanket slows water loss, so garlic continues to draw. The mix under that cover stays loose and workable instead of baking into a brick.

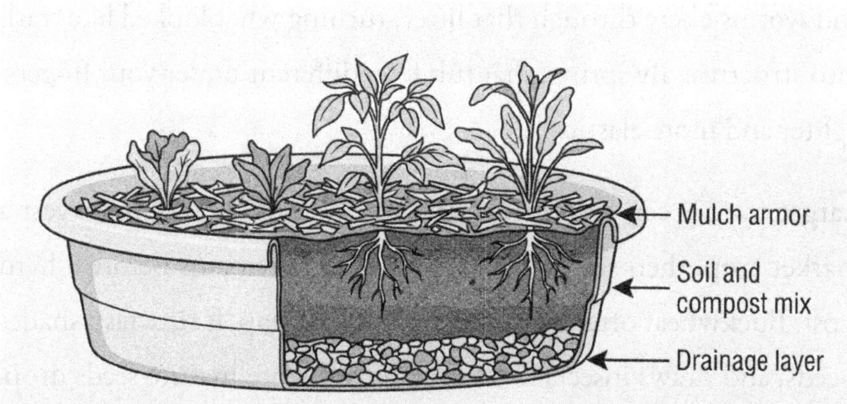

Kiddie Pool, Fabric Bed, or Pot Garden – Layer Cross-Section

When the garlic comes out, the shield does not leave with it. The chopped tops and straw stay in place or get lightly stirred in. Those containers do not head to storage. They shift into the next rotation. A summer crop or new herb moves into the same pool as soon as possible. Sometimes the next act is a heat loving herb like basil or oregano. Sometimes it is a compact vegetable ready to use the loosened, rich mix. The key move stays the same. The surface rarely sees daylight. One set of roots does its work, and before it leaves, another generation moves in. Armor above, rotation below, all inside the same five foot ring.

Not every vessel holds a formal cover crop. Some tubs support one food crop followed by another, with protection provided by chopped residue rather than a separate sowing. A container might host early onions, then switch to a late herb, then rest under a thick blanket of shredded leaves once frost hits. Even that rest period counts. The surface never sits fully exposed. Wind does not whip away fines. Hard rain does not knock particles loose. Microbes and worms chew through that litter, turning what looked like trash into structure. By spring, that tub feels different under your fingers, lighter and more elastic.

Larger frames can blend both tactics. A gardener might harvest a market crop, then sow a quick cover if time remains before a hard frost. Buckwheat often fills that warm season gap. It rises fast, shades weeds, and draws insects to its blossoms. Before mature seeds drop, you cut it and leave the stalks where they fall. The dead growth forms a loose mat. Below, the roots begin to rot, feeding the underground city. Later in the year, you might switch to cool season covers such as oats or cereal rye. They go in on frames that would otherwise sit empty. Roots hold the matrix over winter. Stubble shields the upper layer from ice and driving rain.

Raised beds reward this thinking even more. They drain fast, which helps in wet spells but can strip moisture and structure when the weather turns dry. Protection from residue or winter covers helps those frames act more like healthy field ground. A thin layer of chopped stalks, shredded leaves, or straw across the top offers shelter without smothering seedlings. If you sow a short cover into that frame, it can grow through the litter, doubling the effect. Roots tie together the lower layer while the blanket guards the skin. When you slice the stand off in spring, those stems add to the shield as new crops slide in.

The pattern inside any rotation stays simple. Heavy feeders pull harder and leave the account a little drained. Deep rooted plants, light feeders, and covers help rebuild by pumping sugars down and drawing minerals up. In an above grade setup, that might look like garlic followed by herbs, or a heavy fruit crop followed by a season where the tub rests under leaf mold and a clover stand. In a frame on the ground, it might mean cabbage, then oats and peas, then carrots. Sequences change. The rule does not. Trade hungry crops with builders to keep the account from hitting zero.

My own approach relies on residue and tight rotations in containers, while many colleagues on larger acreages run full cover stands between their commercial crops. They have watched bare blocks slough away under storms and then watched that damage vanish once armor and covers became standard. Their field results appeared beside my research on industrial food and soil damage in *Poisoned at the Grocery Store*. Both paths pointed in the same direction. Ground that stays covered, fed, and rooted resists time and abuse. Ground left exposed and mined collapses into something that barely deserves the name.

Chapter 9: Black Gold From Trash

Compost That Feeds Beds, Pots, and Your Soil Life

Compost in my house starts at the kitchen sink. A big bowl sits beside the drain and catches almost everything that would otherwise go in the trash. Onion ends, potato peels, carrot tops, apple cores, coffee grounds, eggshells, and stray bites nobody finished all land there. Fridge discoveries join if they still look and smell safe.

The bowl sometimes resembles a failed salad bar, but it saves constant trips outside. Every few days, I dump that mess into a big tub by the door, throw on a dry sprinkle, and later shift the mix into a larger composter. It is lazy, honest, and proves you do not need a perfect kitchen to build powerful compost.

Most people buy bagged mixes and fertilizers, then pay again to haul away leaves, weeds, and kitchen scraps. That stream looks normal until you see what it holds. Every trash bag full of plant pieces carries stolen minerals and carbon your ground could have kept. Composting flips that flow. Peelings, stalks, and old leaves turn into dark, crumbly matter that can outdo many store blends and feed a garden for years, not weeks.

Compost is just controlled rot with air. Microbes get a pile of plant scraps, some moisture, some structure, and enough oxygen so the mass never slumps into slime. Dry, carbon rich inputs like old leaves, straw, shredded cardboard, and paper are the browns. Wet, nitrogen rich bits like kitchen peelings, coffee grounds, and fresh grass are the greens. Stack them in loose layers, keep things as damp as a wrung out sponge, and let the tiny livestock work. Done right, the heap heats and shrinks, then cools into something that smells like a forest floor, not a dumpster.

My big workhorses are pallet bins. Four salvaged pallets, nailed together, form a tall, airy box standing on earth. All season long, weeds, stalks, leaves, and material from that sink bowl land there in layers. I do not turn those heaps as often as the manuals suggest. Life and writing steal time. Even without perfect turning, each bin sinks as microbes chew through the load. Every top up stokes the decay fire again. Over months, rough heaps shrink into a deep, dark mass. When the last coarse pieces vanish and the smell turns sweet and earthy, I shovel that treasure out to feed beds and containers.

I also keep a slow, "cold" compost going in larger empty vessels. Some fifty gallon tubs sit around my garden as catch basins for daily waste. Pulled weeds, prunings, and spare trimmings go straight in. A light sprinkle of soil or dried leaves over each new addition keeps flies and odors down. As the level drops, I add more. These slow digesters never blaze, yet they turn light green waste into heavier, more fertile growing media. Later, I scoop the finished layer into productive pots or use it as a top dressing in bigger pools. They act like movable compost mines scattered between crops.

The ground around my containers works as an open air nursery. Many sit on landscape fabric or other barrier material in paths. Feet, sun, and shovels tear that fabric, punching ragged gaps. Those spots lie over sand and native dirt, and I often toss pulled weeds or spilled mix right there. Uprooted weeds dry in the open air. Spilled soil does not worry me. Those scars become test beds instead of eyesores.

After years of this, free crops began to appear in those ragged zones. Seed sifts out of compost, falls from spent plants, or blows in from nearby beds. It drops into the mix of spilled soil and dried weeds, waiting for cool, damp weather. Early in spring, tiny seedlings push through torn fabric and dead stalks. I let them grow just long enough to identify each one. Many of my best chamomile plants came from this waste ground nursery. They sprouted beside the tubs, and I lifted them with a trowel into real containers. In other years, I have found beans, squash, mustard, collards, and more rising from that thrown together mulch. It behaves like a free nursery running on leftovers.

That same fabric zone also grows weeds that I want back on my side. When invaders steal nutrients and water through those tears and seams, they are drawing from the soil and from compost that washed down. I do not see that as a total loss. A weed is a nutrient wrapped in a stem and leaves. If I pull it before seed sets and send it to a pallet bin or a large composter, that stolen wealth comes home. The thief becomes fuel for next year's soil instead of a permanent robber. The catch is timing. Leave weeds alone for three hot weeks in summer, and some will stretch, seed, and take over. Then the free nursery becomes a real problem.

One season showed how fast that can happen. A two week flu lined up with other demands, and I ignored part of my garden. By the time I walked the rows again, weeds had swallowed thirty percent of the space. That patch turned into a jungle, taking hours and days to reclaim. Garlic beds, containers, paths, and compost zones all slipped the leash. Growing, like everything else, remains an experiment lived inside a limited lifetime. Some years punch you. You salvage what you can to the compost and trust yourself to do better on the next round.

Good compost does not need to stink or attract rodents. Fresh kitchen scraps vanish under a layer of browns every time they hit the heap. That cap traps moisture and odor and hides food from scavengers. Meat, large bones, and greasy foods stay out of my outdoor systems. When a bin smells sharp or sour, the usual cause is too much green and not enough air. A quick fork to fluff the top and an extra dose of dry leaves or shredded cardboard bring it back in line. Small shakes of baking soda can tame borderline smells on lids and rims, but air and carbon rich cover remain the real cures.

Not every home has room for pallet bins. Smaller yards and patios can still play. A simple plastic or metal container placed on the ground can hold a family's kitchen scraps and yard waste. Worm bins can run in a corner or even indoors, where red wigglers turn chopped scraps into fine castings. Some people use half buried buckets with drilled holes as in bed digesters. Scraps go in, lids go on, and worms and microbes pull breakdown products out through the holes into nearby soil. Every version follows the same law: browns, greens, air, and moisture, set up to rot in your favor instead of in a landfill.

The line between compost pile and garden often disappears. In a raised frame, you can dig shallow trenches between rows and bury cooled kitchen scraps and soft waste. The bed becomes the bin. Microbes and worms handle the breakdown, and roots later chase the nutrients they leave behind. Some of my above grade containers spend part of the year as mini digesters, packed with layers of leaves and soft debris, capped with a little soil or straw. By the next planting, those layers slump into something close to a new potting mix. That material later supports garlic, herbs, or the next round of vegetables in the same vessel.

Not every scrap belongs in these systems. Oily foods, large chunks of meat or cheese, glossy colored paper, and anything treated with the same poisons I worried about in *Poisoned at the Grocery Store* stay out. Compost multiplies whatever you feed it. Good inputs give rich, safe humus. Contaminated ones can carry residues into your ground and onto your plate. When in doubt, I hand suspect bits to municipal trash and protect the integrity of my home heaps.

Finished compost announces itself by feel and smell. It turns dark, crumbly, and cool to the touch. Recognizable stems, rinds, and leaves vanish. The whole mass smells like a forest floor after rain. That is when it leaves the pallet bin or big tub and heads back to production. I spread it as a shallow skin over beds, blend it into my own potting mixes, or tuck it around heavy feeders as a slow side dressing. It adds structure, water holding, and life more than raw fertilizer punch. Paired with the armor and rotations from the last chapter, this black gold turns tired dirt into a steady engine.

Some gardeners take this even further, building raised beds with a compost core that eats kitchen scraps and feeds itself. The next chapter steps into that idea and shows how a pattern born in drought can break the raised bed habit of buying bags forever.

Chapter 10: Keyhole Gardens – Self Feeding Beds That Break the System

Compost Cores, Less Water, More Control

This chapter shows how to turn a raised bed into a self feeding system so you buy fewer inputs and depend less on anyone's supply chain but your own. Keyhole designs turn trash and rinse water into a steady food supply.

Every spring, big box stores count on you to fail. People line up for bags of "premium" mix and bright fertilizer, dumping over a hundred dollars into each wooden frame before a single seed hits the dirt. Those boxes look neat and modern, but they are built hungry by design. They slump, dry out, and starve plants until you drag your cart back for another round of material and chemicals. That is not an accident.

I had to add this idea to the book because it fits everything we have talked about. I have seen keyhole gardens in use and read a great deal about them. I want to be clear up front. I have not built a classic stone ring myself, but I do run smaller versions in large above ground containers that follow the same science.

Across drought stricken hills in places like Zimbabwe and Lesotho, families facing failed rains and empty wallets had to answer a brutal question. How do you grow food when you cannot buy fertilizer, cannot haul endless water, and sometimes cannot even stand long enough to tend a field? Out of that crisis, aid workers and local farmers rebuilt the idea of a growing space from the ground up. They created something that should make every Western gardener stop and stare. A waist high circle of rubble wrapped around a compost filled heart that runs on kitchen scraps and almost no water. They call it the keyhole garden.

Earlier in this book, we walked through framed beds, healing mounds, above ground pools, and big pots. Those systems already move you away from flat, dead lawns toward ground that can recover. Keyhole layouts push the idea one step further. Rather than feeding plots from a pile off to the side, they place a compost core right in the middle of the action and let roots eat from the inside out.

Picture a rough circle six to eight feet across, built from whatever the site gives you. Fieldstones, broken bricks, bottles packed into clay, stacked up to your waist so an older gardener can harvest without bending. From above, it looks like a clock face with one slice missing.

That wedge is the walkway you use to reach the interior. In that opening stands the engine of the system, a simple mesh basket just wide enough for your arm, sunk into the mix and lined with sticks and dry grass.

Into that tube goes everything your trash can usually hides. Banana peels, coffee grounds, eggshells, torn cardboard, and a handful of dry leaves on top to keep things decent. Every time someone rinses a dish or dumps a pot of clean rinse water, it goes through that core. Rather than splashing across the surface and vanishing, the water sinks through layers of scraps. It dissolves nutrients as it moves and pushes them outward like veins feeding a body. In field use, these compost heart beds can be watered as little as once a week in the dry season, using far less than conventional plots that gulp and waste every bucket.

Many of us already compost kitchen scraps, but we often do it in a heap or bin far from the main growing rows. This approach keeps that energy in one tight spot in the middle of the planting zone, where roots can find it faster. You do not have to copy the African stone circles to use the idea. Dropping a simple mesh cylinder into a framed bed or a very large pot follows the same science. Feed that core, water it through, and let the planting area become its own stomach. As I keep saying, your garden is your experiment. Some of my larger setups already work this way in a small form.

The result is a quiet kind of shock. In regions where home plots had shriveled into dust, tens of thousands of these circles sprang up. Years later, many were still in use, still feeding families long after the aid trucks vanished. Raise the organic matter in poor ground by a few percent, and the moisture holding capacity can jump several times over. Brittle sand turns into a sponge that stays damp long after the sun should have baked it dry. Rather than watching fertility wash away, each watering becomes an infusion of life aimed right at the root zone.

Beneath the surface, that "mess" of scraps becomes a working engine. Earthworms slip in and out of the core like tiny plows. They shred peels, drag particles outward, and leave castings richer than most products on the shelf. Microbes swarm the pile, breaking it down with such intensity that they generate heat. That warmth can nudge the surrounding mix a few degrees higher. In cool highlands, farmers noticed their keyhole plots stayed frost free longer, squeezing extra weeks of harvest out of a season that used to quit early.

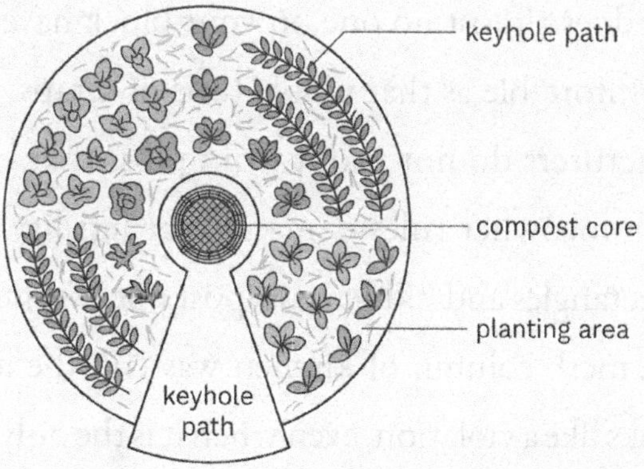

Think about that for a moment. While millions of Western gardeners reload subscription kits that never feed themselves, a cheap roll of mesh and a season's worth of kitchen scraps can turn almost any box into a self feeding machine that refuses to die. The only real input is your daily life. Peel potatoes, make coffee, crack eggs, tear junk mail. Drop it into the core, dust with dry leaves or shredded paper, and walk away. Worms and microbes work harder than you ever will, day and night, without a paycheck, without a hose, without a label.

On my own counter, a bowl next to the sink collects all vegetable scraps and trimmings. That bowl is not garbage. It is future energy for the plants. I do not have the space to stack full keyhole rings in my small yard. What I can do, and what you can do, is make smaller mesh cylinders, stuff them with scraps, and set them inside large frames and big tubs. It is the same idea at a different scale. You adapt the method to your space rather than waiting for perfect conditions that never come.

So why does almost no one on your block have one? The answer is as uncomfortable as that visible tube of scraps. Garden centers and manufacturers do not profit from plots that can feed themselves. Many homeowner rules demand that fertility stay invisible. Neat cedar rectangles and hidden compost piles fit the picture of a "good" yard. A mesh column of kitchen waste in the middle of a planting area looks like a violation, even when it is the only part of the property actually doing real work. We traded living cycles for clean lines and then wondered why our rows behave like expensive ornaments rather than survival tools.

You do not need a crisis, a charity, or a plane ticket to build a self feeding layout. You can drop a compost core into almost any framed space or large container you already own. Take a roll of chicken mesh and bend it into a cylinder about 12 inches across and 2 to 3 feet tall. Dig a shallow hole in the center of the bed, line it with small sticks to keep water moving, and set the tube in place so it rises slightly above the mix. Fill it, layer by layer, with raw vegetable scraps and dry material. No meat, no dairy, no greasy cooked leftovers. If you can, toss in a handful of worms as if you are seeding the future.

Around that core, plant in loose rings. Thirsty leafy crops such as lettuce and spinach grow closer to the tube. Tougher plants and herbs sit toward the edges. Each time you water, aim for the center. Each time you cook, feed the core first. Over weeks, the contents will slump as they digest. The structure will settle, and you will top it up with more scraps or a decent mix. That slow sinking is not failure. It is proof that your plot is eating, growing, and turning waste into harvest.

The payoff is not subtle. Self feeding circles like these often yield noticeably more than boxes that rely only on store bought inputs. Greens stand taller. Roots drive deeper. The ground under your feet turns dark, loose, and alive instead of pale, compacted, and exhausted. What began as a strange, "messy" column becomes a quiet ritual that closes the loop between the kitchen and the yard. You stop being only a consumer of products and promises. You become the caretaker of a miniature ecosystem that pays you back every day.

In a world of rising food prices and shrinking water tables, depending on disposable growing solutions is not just expensive. It is dangerous. The keyhole idea, born in some of the harshest conditions on earth, exposes a truth that should feel almost scandalous to anyone who has ever pushed a loaded cart through a garden center. Nature never stopped working for free. The only question is whether you will keep feeding a hungry box that needs rescue every spring, or build a living bed that feeds itself and you season after season.

The next chapter moves from self feeding structures to water capture and storage, so the moisture that lands on your property also starts working full time for you.

Chapter 11: Water Capture and Drought Defense

Free Rain, Tight Rows, and Backup Plans for Dry Spells

Gardens rarely fail from lack of ideas. They fail due to a lack of water. A rich bed and perfect layout still collapse when the sky shuts off for three weeks, and the hose cannot keep up. One space with barrels, tight alleys, and stored water limps through a dry spell. Another, with exposed dirt and no reserves, cooks to dust. In a world that feels less stable each year, water becomes the real gatekeeper between a hopeful grower and a dead patch.

Rain still falls for free, but water bills and rules do not. Many places now warn, meter, or restrict how much water you can use on lawns and gardens in a drought. Some regions even write strange limits on how much roof runoff you can hold or direct into storage, often to protect larger water rights systems.

Details change by state and city, but the message stays the same. You cannot assume endless cheap city water or full freedom to run huge tanks without checking your local code. That pushes every gardener toward experiments. You learn where you can follow the rules, where you can work inside them, and how to keep crops alive even when the official system does not make sense.

My above-grade setup does not look like the spaced-out catalog beds in glossy videos. I push pots and pools into close ranks, with rims almost touching. Those narrow lanes capture more storm water. When a downpour hits, water runs off one container into the next instead of disappearing into wide, dry paths.

Tight spacing also shades the walls. When rows sit too far apart, the sun blasts every exposed side and bakes the mix inside. Closer bands still allow light to reach foliage, but the walls stay cooler and lose less moisture. It is not a tidy magazine look. It is a survival layout.

Empty buckets act as quiet allies. I scatter several five-gallon pails among the containers. When it rains, they fill. When I run the overhead sprinklers because there is no time to hand-water every pot, they fill again. Sprinklers are not ideal. They can wet leaves and encourage disease on tomatoes, cucumbers, and other susceptible crops.

Yet this is not a perfect world. Work, illness, or sudden heat waves sometimes force blunt tools. I call the extra disease risk from those rushed sprinkler runs collateral garden damage. The key is to claw value back. Those full buckets sit right beside thirsty roots. I paid for that sprayed water on the meter, so I dip it out later and pour it at the base where it does real work.

More careful systems run when time allows. Some lines carry simple drip or trickle tubing near plant crowns. Timers take over when I cannot stand there with a hose. They bring their own quirks and failures, so I never install as much as I imagine. Life cuts those plans down. Even partial coverage helps. A section with drip saves time and water, leaving more energy to spot-water the rest or haul buckets where they matter most. Overhead sprinklers step in only when everything else falls behind, not as my first choice.

Larger storage still earns its space. Several 55-gallon drums sit under gutters or near roof edges. When a solid storm hits, they fill fast. That cache waits for the next dry stretch, when hoses and municipal pressure might be costly or limited. Years ago, I pushed this further while renting a greenhouse on a remote farm. A runoff pond sat about 300 feet away.

Once a week, I pumped water from that pond, filled fourteen drums, then pushed it back into the greenhouse tanks and lines. It worked, but taught another lesson. Greenhouses bring their own headaches. Deer and groundhogs chew through plastic and chew up seedlings. Summer heat under film can kill as fast as frost. The learning curve and upkeep felt like a second career. I walked away from that book and left greenhouse life to someone with a greater appetite for that world.

All this hardware still sits on one rule. Your deepest tank is the ground itself. A living, well-fed profile can hold a huge volume between storms. Organic matter and good structure make it a sponge rather than a brick. The compost and armor from earlier chapters feed that structure, but they never store a drop if water never reaches them. Every barrel, bucket, and improvised catch rig buys time. Every tight row and shaded container wall slows loss. Every drip line and careful bucket pour directs water to roots instead of into the air and pavement.

Drought still arrives. Forecasts still lie. When weeks pass with no rain and limits tighten, you shift from comfort watering to triage. Deep-rooted perennials, long-lived herbs, and key seed parents get the closest care. Quick crops already near harvest may get less. Some sections may be allowed to fade so others live. Old sheets, tarps, or shade-cloth scraps can stretch across rows during the hottest hours, reducing stress even when water remains scarce. You will lose some plants. Call it collateral garden damage and move forward instead of quitting.

My setup, with its tight ranks, mismatched buckets, improvised drums, and occasional emergency sprinkler run, will never win a beauty prize. It is not built for drone shots. It is built to keep roots alive long enough to feed me when the weather and systems turn strange.

Many of my colleagues on larger ground carry the same mindset into bigger tanks, more formal drip layouts, and ponds designed for irrigation. Their work shows that catch, store, and slow use beats wishful thinking every time. Your version might be one barrel and four buckets on a balcony rail. It still counts.

Every drop you capture and aim on purpose is one less drop you beg from a fragile system that can shut off without warning. The next chapter shifts back below the surface, focusing on how living roots and cover crops hold that captured water in place rather than letting it run off to the nearest ditch.

Chapter 12: Smart Rotation, Less Disease

Moving Plant Families to Starve Pests and Blights

Some gardens crash because the same crops keep landing in the same place. Tomatoes, peppers, or cabbage sit in one bed year after year, and each season the plants look weaker, bugs arrive earlier, and blights hit harder. Another space shuffles plant families and sees fewer disasters. Soil remembers what you grow. It rewards variety and punishes repetition with a slow rise of pests and diseases that treat your beds like an endless buffet.

Crop rotation sounds fancy, but it means one move. Change where each crop family grows from year to year so no bed or pot feeds the same enemy on a fixed schedule. Many insects and pathogens are picky eaters. Tomato problems target the nightshade clan. Clubroot loves the mustard clan. Serve their favorite meal in the same slot every time, and they explode. Move that meal and their life cycle breaks, numbers fall, and your space starts to feel like yours again.

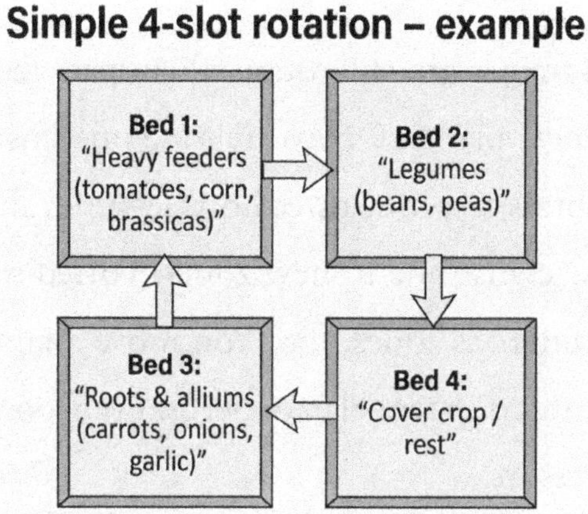

Move plant families, not just crops, each year.

Families matter more than individual names. Tomatoes, peppers, eggplant, and potatoes all sit in the nightshade group and share soil borne diseases and chewing foes. Cabbage, broccoli, kale, collards, mustard, and radishes belong to the brassica group and share problems such as clubroot and certain wilts. Beans and peas share the legume clan, partner with nitrogen fixing bacteria on their roots, and can pass some root troubles along if never moved. You do not need a botany degree. You need a short list of which crops travel together and a habit of not parking that group in the same earth over and over.

One rule does most of the work. After you grow a heavy, disease prone family in one spot, let that area rest from that clan for at least three years. Nightshades like tomatoes do best on a three year loop. Brassicas often need three or more years, especially where clubroot or wilt has shown up. Legumes can come back sooner, around two years, because their soil issues build more slowly. Longer breaks help, yet short shifts matter. Moving tomatoes one bed over beats planting them on last year's root zone.

Small yards and frames can still rotate when space feels tight. Think in zones, not single plants. One year, zone one hosts nightshades; zone two hosts brassicas; zone three hosts legumes and light feeders. Next year, those clans slide to new zones. Potted setups can treat groups of containers as zones, too. You move a family out of one cluster and slide in a different clan or herbs. Even loose, approximate rotation cuts pressure.

My own path shows how rotation sometimes arrives sideways. One year, whiteflies tore through a past container layout. The invasion likely rode in on nursery stock and did not care about my plans. It wrecked about seventy five percent of that garden despite sprays, traps, and every trick I threw at it. The move that worked felt brutal. I cut tomatoes from about half the space, down to maybe ten percent, and filled the freed vessels with herbs.

That shift yanked me into a new level. Now I grow and dry more than twenty five herbs and grind them into evening teas and kitchen blends, which deserve their own book. Whitefly pressure faded once its favorite hosts thinned out, and I learned to be far more careful with plugs and auction plants. Many neighbors quit after their own infestations. A bad year hurts, but it is not a verdict. You come back sharper.

I do not run a strict, chart driven rotation. My above grade world behaves differently. Many vessels stay married to certain herbs that return year after year. I often leave empty containers alone until mid spring to see what volunteers. Free food rises when you give it a chance. Some seasons, sage surged in two tubs. I dried so much that I skipped planting sage the next year and used that slot for something else. Chamomile, lemon balm, and mint also return home. Those three form the backbone of many daily tea mixes. They earn their space, so they stay.

Containers provide a quiet form of rotation, with crops on top that look familiar. When I flip, refill, or top up pots with compost and fresh mix, the microscopic world changes. Some disease pressure dilutes. Moving containers to new spots in the tight rows also shifts sun, wind, and moisture patterns around the roots. I still avoid dropping the same touchy family into the same tired mix year after year, yet I keep productive perennial herbs in place. Over time, as the garden settles, more food appears as volunteers and carryovers. The job becomes guiding and editing the returning cast instead of starting from bare soil every spring.

Rotation does not erase every problem, but it pairs well with earlier tools. Cover crops and compost help rebuild structure and biology, yet some pathogens linger in residues and in the thin film around roots. Moving plant families away from those hot spots gives the underground life time to outcompete leftover trouble. Strong, diverse biology from your compost and mulch then works on a different set of crops instead of fighting the same war all the time. You build a double shield without reaching for harsh chemicals.

Common problems and system moves

Problem	System move that helps
Soil dries out fast in heat	Deep mulch armor, fewer shallow waterings, more roots
Heavy rain pounds beds	Keep soil covered, add cover crops, use shallow basins
Early blight on tomatoes	Rotate out of bed, increase mulch, trim lower leaves
Root crops split or rot	Improve drainage, avoid overwatering, loosen soil
Beds crust after storms	No bare soil, keep residue on top, avoid deep tilling
Yields drop each year	Add compost/'black gold', rotate families, add cover

Perfect charts are optional. Mindset matters. You notice patterns. You remember which clan sat where, even if only roughly. You listen when a crop starts failing in one bed and give that spot a break. You stay ready to pivot, like after my whitefly year, when reality punched a hole in my plan. Some colleagues with larger plots map rotations years ahead and track clear drops in pest and disease pressure over time. My version stays looser, more like steering a river of pots and herbs than managing straight rows. Both prove the same thing. Ground that sees variety stays kinder. Ground that sees the same act on repeat pushes back.

Rotation, in the end, is one more way to think a few seasons ahead instead of only thinking about next weekend. Healthy soil, stored water, and smart movement of plant families work together. They turn a garden from a fragile, one year gamble into a long game that can take a bad season, a pest flare, or a surprise blight and still stand back up.

Chapter 13: Underground Livestock

Microbes, Worms, and the Soil Food Web

Most people still call it dirt, as if it were dead. Healthy soil is closer to a crowded city. A single handful can hold more living creatures than there are people on this planet. They move, eat, fight, and trade under your feet while you stand there thinking you see brown stuff.

Dead, pale, compacted ground that grows little but weeds belongs more on a construction site. Dark, crumbly, worm filled soil that smells like a forest after rain belongs in a garden. Every step in this book has been about feeding that hidden livestock, not about feeding tomatoes or garlic.

The underground cast looks small, yet it runs everything. Bacteria and fungi sit at the base of this web. They cover root hairs, leaf bits, and compost flakes and chew them into smaller pieces. As they work, they convert nitrogen and other elements into forms plants can use and lock them inside their own bodies. Protozoa and many nematodes graze on those microbes and release nutrients back into the soil solution when they eat, pee, and die. Tiny arthropods like mites and springtails shred plant debris into confetti, giving bacteria and fungi more surfaces to attack. Larger creatures, such as earthworms, pull all of this deeper, grind it, and mix it into the soil's mineral skeleton.

Plants do not sit there waiting for whatever happens. Their roots hire help. During photosynthesis, plants absorb carbon dioxide and use sunlight to produce sugars. They spend a surprising share of those sugars underground. Roots leak out a mix of sugars, acids, and other compounds into the thin zone around them called the rhizosphere. Those leaks act like paychecks for microbes. Certain bacteria and fungi gather to eat those exudates. In return, they mine locked up nutrients from organic matter, clay, and rock particles and return them to the plant at the root surface. Fungal partners called mycorrhizae grow long threads from the roots out into the soil. Those threads act like a second root system, hauling in water and minerals from far beyond the reach of the plant's own tips. Think of roots as shop owners. They pay their security and delivery crews in sugar. Those crews keep the shelves stocked and kick out troublemakers before they reach the front door.

Earthworms deserve their own wanted poster. Their tunnels act like four wheel drive tillers that never need gas. As they push through soil, they loosen and aerate it, allowing roots and air to move deeper. Water follows those channels downward instead of sheeting off the surface. Soils with plenty of worms can drain several times faster than similar soils without them, yet also hold more moisture once the water sinks in. Worms drag leaves, compost, and other organic matter down their burrows, grind it, and coat their tunnel walls with casts rich in nutrients and stable organic glues. Those casts often contain several times more available phosphorus, potassium, calcium, and nitrogen than the surrounding bulk soil and help cement particles into crumbs that resist erosion yet absorb water. Roots find and line these worm corridors because they offer the easiest path and the richest food.

You do not need a microscope to know whether this underground herd is waking up. Healthy soil looks darker, often like chocolate or coffee grounds, compared with the nearby pale, tired dirt. It crumbles between your fingers when moist instead of breaking into hard clods or dust. It smells rich and earthy, not sour, rotten, or chemical. That scent comes from compounds such as geosmin made by soil bacteria. When you dig a small hole, you should see worms, tiny insects, and sometimes fine white fungal threads spread through the soil, not bare grains. One simple test many soil people use is to dig a square about a foot wide and a foot deep, tip it on a tarp, and count worms. Ten or more in that block hints at good biology. Fewer suggests that your underground herd still needs to be built.

Some habits flatten this whole system. Repeated deep tilling chops fungal networks and worm tunnels into smaller pieces, leaving organisms exposed to heat, air, and predators. Heavy doses of harsh, salt based fertilizers over time can stress sensitive microbes and push the soil toward dependence on fresh bags rather than its own biology. Broad spectrum fungicides and soil sterilizers do not always distinguish between pathogens and helpful fungi. They can wipe out protective guilds along with the troublemakers you aimed at. Constant bare soil bakes and erodes the very habitat this herd needs. Each of these shortcuts might fix a short term issue while raising the long term cost underfoot.

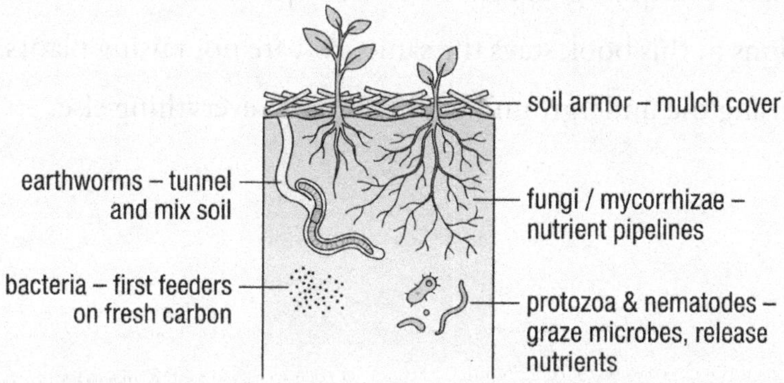

Underground livestock – the herd under your mulch

I have seen the difference in my own beds and pots. Places where I once fought concrete soil now take a spade after a few years of gentle handling, organic matter, and no deep disturbance. Worms show up in the shovel full instead of hiding somewhere below. Containers that used to crust over and crack between watering's now hold their shape, drain without drowning, and keep roots moist longer once their soil has time to turn from tired mix into something closer to real earth.

Those changes did not come from a single product. They came from feeding and protecting the underground livestock long enough for them to rebuild their city.

Once you see soil as a living community instead of as dead dirt, every choice in the garden carries a new weight. You still care about pounds of tomatoes and bulbs of garlic, yet you also care about whether the microbes and worms want to come back for another shift. When they thrive, plants root deeper, handle stress better, and resist disease more naturally. The quiet goal behind the beds, pots, mulch, compost, and rotations in this book stays the same. You are not raising plants. You are raising the underground herd that raises everything else.

Chapter 14: Seed Saving and True Independence

Keeping Your Own Heirloom Seed Bank

Store racks look full until the wrong year hits. In 2020, some stores had almost no seed. Panic buying, supply glitches, or one bad season at a seed farm can wipe out favorites overnight. The gardener who trusts only those hooks stares at bare metal. The gardener with jars and envelopes in a closet plans the next planting. Holding seed means holding next year's food, and the year after, in your own hands.

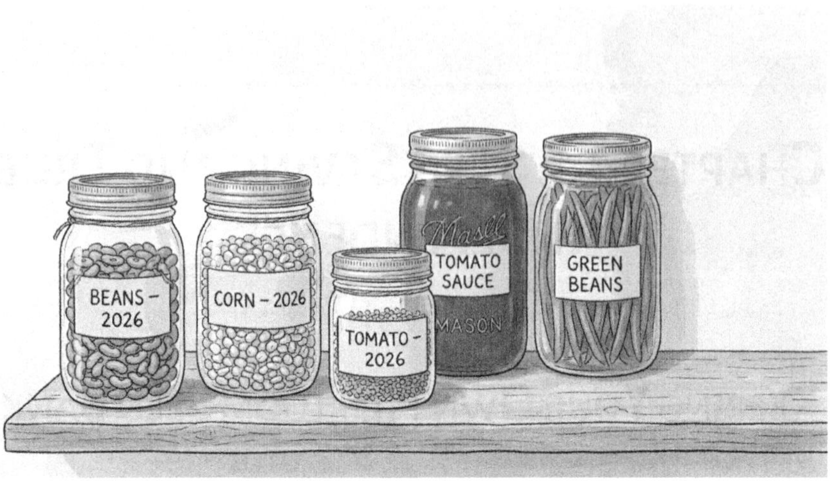

I once grew tiny orange sweet peppers that tasted like candy. They were hybrids and could not truly reproduce. I bought fresh packets every year. In 2024, they vanished. Something went wrong at the company, and the line disappeared from the catalogs. I found substitutes, but the exact favorite was gone. We live in a world with too wide a variety of paper and not enough control in our own hands.

Not every packet behaves the same. Heirloom and other open pollinated lines give offspring close to the parent as long as they do not cross with different kinds. A good red paste tomato can keep its shape and flavor when you save the best fruits. Hybrids play a different game. They come from a planned cross built for one season of performance. Saved hybrid seed often throws weak, odd plants, or nothing at all. Scoop out seeds from a supermarket cucumber, dry them, and plant them, and you might get bitter vines, stunted plants, or a tangle that never fruits. Commercial melons, peppers, and squash often behave similarly. Those shelves sell food, not genetics. I avoid hybrids when I can because they choke off real savings and keep you buying the same line every year.

Some crops are easy gates into this world. Beans and peas mostly pollinate themselves inside their flowers before insects ever arrive. Many older tomatoes do the same, with modest blossoms that keep pollen close. Lettuce stays true if you are not crowding many strains shoulder to shoulder. These crops let you save without fretting over stray pollen. A few plants, left to finish their cycle, can fill jars with enough seed for several years. When hot weather hits and my lettuce bolts, I let a few stalks stand and go to seed. They look shaggy and wild, yet they carry next year's salads in those fluff topped heads.

The steps do not need a lab. Pick strong plants, not runts or sickly stems. Let at least one stand per species go all the way to mature seed, or mark a few top fruits and pods and let them fully ripen and dry. Harvest at the right stage. Separate the seed from thc pulp or chaff. Dry it in shade with good air until it feels hard, not rubbery. Only then does it go into containers. That simple path works for many home staples.

My own stash grew from habits, not charts. Everything lives inside a big latching tub so it stays together and avoids sudden humidity swings. Inside, seeds ride in whatever works. Old prescription vials block light and snap shut. Glass and plastic jars hold larger amounts. Paper packets and envelopes tuck between them for small runs and new arrivals. The bin looks more like a junk drawer than a catalog, yet it shelters years of genetics.

Out in the beds and tubs, I try to give each species at least one parent. A basil that shrugs off heat, a parsley that laughs at frost, a lettuce that stays crisp, a tomato that tastes better than its peers all earn the right to carry the line. Each year, I also pull in a few new heirlooms from outside. Some come from seed houses. Some come from small growers. Once, I bought dandelion seed for fat roots and dried those roots for tea experiments. Another year, I walked into an Amish hardware store and walked out with old lines you never see in glossy catalogs. Everything ends back in the same master tub, waiting for a turn in the soil.

Not every crop deserves the space in my above grade world. I write this book for regular gardeners, not for corn breeders. I do not grow corn or sunflowers in my containers. They steal too much light from shorter pots and crowd my tight rows. I would gladly line a front yard with sunflowers, but many cities and neighbors still prefer short, green, useless grass. They choose a thirsty carpet over living food and seed.

Purity matters more for some crops than others. Corn and many brassicas cross freely, and traits blur if different strains flower side by side. If you care about keeping a line true, keep only one kind for seed in a given year, or separate cousins by distance, barriers, or timing so their bloom does not overlap. In a smaller space, the easiest move is simple. One sweet corn for seed this year, one kale strain next year, one radish after that. You keep the work simple and the lines clean.

Storage keeps all that effort from dying on a shelf. Seed wants three things to stay alive yet quiet: cool, dark, and dry. Every container gets a label with its name, year, and a note such as "early," "hot," or "from volunteer." The big box lives in a steady, cooler corner away from sunlight and furnace blasts. Most seeds hold decent germination for several years under those conditions. That slow fade becomes a feature once you stay in motion. Each season, you plant some, save some, and push the line forward.

There are tradeoffs. As seeds age, germination drops. One hundred percent germination—every seed sprouting—is almost impossible. Maybe the first year, a packet of heirloom tomatoes gives eighty sprouts out of one hundred. Eight years later, you might see only twenty. Some growers freeze part of their seed stash to slow this slide. Cold storage can stretch life, but moisture control becomes critical. If a seed goes into a freezer with too much water, ice crystals tear living cells. If it goes in very dry and sealed, it can stay viable far longer than it would at room temperature. The world's largest backup, the Svalbard Global Seed Vault in the Arctic, uses deep cold and stable rock to safeguard thousands of food lines in case entire regions fail.

Archaeologists sometimes find ancient seeds in tombs and buried jars. A few very dry, well stored grains and beans have sprouted after hundreds or even thousands of years. Those stories are rare, but they prove a point. With the right care, tiny flecks of life can outlive empires.

Saving does not have to stay a solo sport. Local swaps, church basement trades, and friend circles let growers move extra seed and rare finds. One person might keep a bean that climbs hard in the wind. Another preserves a pepper that sets fruit in a short, cold summer. Trading those envelopes spreads risk and keeps more varieties alive even when catalogs quietly drop them. In a shaky world, a small ring of gardeners swapping paper at a hardware counter can protect more food security than a polished brochure.

I tend to drink from the half empty glass, so I overbuild my safety net. I collect seeds from multiple sources. In my beds, I allow certain overripe fruits and vegetables to fall and rot in place. If I do not flip an above ground pot, sometimes a surprise rises there in spring. I gather seed heads and pods when I can. The worst that happens is this: I forget to label them, and three months later, I cannot recall the exact type. I also raid store racks at the end of the season when prices drop by eighty percent. Those packets may not be the freshest, yet many still sprout. In February, I visit Amish seed houses and hardware counters and buy the brands local growers trust. Then I indulge myself and order a few strange, fun things from small outfits online.

You can picture the result. My seed container is about four feet long, twenty inches wide, and fourteen inches deep. It is packed with bags, jars, packets, and even some vacuum sealed bundles. I have enough to plant ten versions of my current layout. If I ever had to bug out because of a nearby nuclear accident, that seed box would be one of the first things in the car.

Over time, all these efforts gather. Volunteers that pop up in ground fabric tears or old tubs become part of the living bank. A tough chamomile that germinates in a scrap zone and survives neglect earns a real home and later a labeled jar. A lemon balm that shrugs off heat becomes mother to many tea plants. I do not rush to rip out greenery along my walkways where soil and torn fabric meet. Many of those "weeds" are old friends in new spots. I lift them, move them into real containers, and let them join the next generation of seed parents.

Seed saving closes the loop in a way no store ever will. You are no longer just feeding this year's garden. You are quietly stocking future seasons, one dried pod and scribbled label at a time.

Chapter 15: From Poisoned Store to Home Grown Plate

Building Your Personal Food Safety System

Food in many stores and restaurants has been unsafe for a long time. Fryers never rest, oils go rancid, mystery sauces hide old ingredients, and chemicals and pesticides ride every plate. I wrote whole books about poison on menus and in grocery aisles, but this book walks the other side of that line. Here, you raise food for daily meals and long term storage so you do not depend on strangers and supply chains for every bite.

Home preservation stretches a short harvest into a long eating window. I am not talking about someone with a bunker of dusty cans they will never touch. Freezing, dehydrating, water bath canning, and pressure canning all have roles. Freezing keeps flavor and texture closest to fresh and works well for many fruits, vegetables, and cooked dishes. The cost hides in electricity and space. A packed chest freezer in the basement depends on a single compressor, a single breaker, and a single power connection, all of which can fail without warning.

Drying shrinks food into light, shelf stable pieces that fit in jars and bags. Done at a lower heat, it keeps much of the nutrition, but the texture changes; some slices go leathery, others crisp. Water bath canning serves the high acid world: pickles, jams, jellies, and many tomato products. Boiling water for the proper time kills microbes and gives shelf stable jars, but this method cannot safely handle low acid foods. Pressure canning takes low acid vegetables, meats, and full meals to higher temperatures under steam. Done by the book, it gives years of safe shelf life.

Done carelessly, it can invite botulism, a nerve poison that can kill from one bad jar. That risk is real enough to demand respect, good gear, and tested recipes, not guesswork or social media shortcuts. Tradeoffs matter more than slogans. Freezing is fast: blanch, cool, pack, stack, and shut the lid. On a chaotic harvest day, the freezer often wins for food you plan to eat within a year. Its weak point is grid failure. One storm, one blown transformer, or one long outage can turn that chest into a warm box of slime if you are not ready to cook or cannot move fast.

Dehydrating sips energy and preserves food you can carry, mail, or stash without fear of a dead outlet or a pinging lid. It shines for herbs, fruits, thin slices, and ingredients you plan to grind into teas or dry mixes. Water bath canning is ideal when you want bright, sweet, or sour jars on the shelf. It is a keeper when you want ready to eat vegetables in glass, not in metal lined with suspect coatings and mystery glue. None of these routes is free. Each one buys distance from shelves you already distrust.

Growing and preserving more food also rewires your yard. Grass stops getting a free ride. Every square foot you convert to beds, tubs, or fruit trees reduces mowing time and fuel use. That patch stops begging for fertilizer and weed killer and starts paying rent in food. Tight ranks of containers catch rainwater instead of sending it to the storm drain. A small front strip planted with kale, herbs, and peppers can cut down on grocery trips and shorten your mowing. Those hours move from pacing behind a roaring mower to trimming beans, loading dehydrator trays, or lining jars on a towel.

The last part of this story belongs to your daily life. A normal week shifts when more meals come from the yard and pantry and fewer from fast food bags and mystery buffets. Breakfast might pull from frozen berries, dry granola, and home canned peaches. Lunch leans on fresh greens, a jar of beans, and a sprinkling of dried herbs. Supper joins pressure canned stew with dehydrated vegetables and a frozen side. Each plate becomes a quiet audit of what you control and what you still buy. You see real tomatoes and real garlic, not flavor sprayed from a bottle. You feel where each part came from instead of trusting a barcode.

At the beginning of this book, we talked about how few people garden now because the system pushes big agriculture and big boxes. The bottom line is harsh. Many commercial products and preserved "foods" built from them do more to keep big pharma busy than to keep you well. We are kept busy with work, screens, and a thousand small wastes of time. If you claw back even a slice of that, you can grow, cultivate, and harvest part of your own diet. No, you cannot keep cows or chickens in most small yards. City codes and tight lots cap how far you can go. Baby steps still matter. A few beds, a row of tubs, or ten jars on a shelf can be a life changer and a slow drop in sickness.

Touching soil pulls you back toward sanity. Digging, turning, and building soil brings you closer to earth than any treadmill ever will. Fresh air, bending and lifting, and quiet thinking between rows work on the body and the mind at once. When you see peppers and tomatoes you raised yourself, it brings satisfaction and comfort that a beach chair and umbrella drink cannot touch. You built those calories from seed instead of swiping plastic at a drive through.

We are taught that life is a two choice world: the right way and the wrong way, store food or no food. The truth sits in between. You do not have to live on jars alone, nor do you have to trust the store alone. Your path might be ground beds, pots, or hydroponic buckets on a balcony. It might be a few herbs under a window or a yard full of fabric covered rows. It will always be an experiment, and you will learn more each season you try.

I might plant twelve hundred cloves of garlic and harvest only seven hundred heads because I laid the straw too deep, or a freeze came bare, or some cloves were never viable. For a whole year, the stores around me were out of the garlic I wanted. Maybe crops failed, maybe shipping broke, maybe rules cut imports; the reasons pile up. When I plant my own saved garlic from the previous season, it still produces. It may not hit 100 percent, but it hits enough that I am not standing under fluorescent lights, hoping a truck shows up.

My garden will never look like a postcard. Something always goes sideways: weather, time, health, or plain bad luck. You will never hit 100 percent optimization either. A "bad" year that gives you half your planned harvest is still fifty percent more food than your neighbor with the perfect green lawn produced. Their yard ate money. Yours fed you.

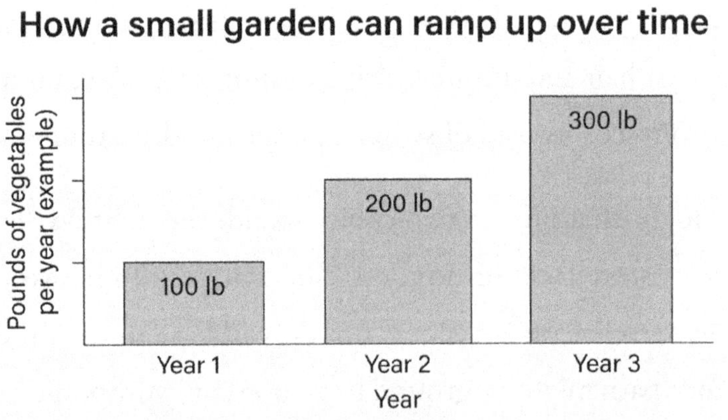

Example ramp based on typical home garden yields - results vary by space, climate, and habits.

Now you know the pieces. Decide what fits your life and your lot: above ground, in ground, greenhouse, or a mix. Build and collect soil. Gather and save seed. Choose preservation methods that match your climate, power situation, and nerves. Maybe you need trellises, cattle panels, or poles for vining crops. Maybe you need drip hoses, or maybe you need to cut a few branches to bring in more light. If you have a forest edge, mushrooms might be your best crop, and you will find a book on logs and spores. If you have a pond, you might route scraps to ducks, raise fish, or net bluegill for the pan.

If you live in a high rise, you may only line one sill with herbs and plant microgreens on a rack. I know people whose entire "garden" is four tomato plants where foundation shrubs used to sit. It is not all or nothing. It is something, and something is where you start.

In a better world, we would grow more plants we can eat or drink and fewer lawns we can only mow. We would trade jars and baskets with neighbors rather than compare riding mowers. For now, that is a dream. The first crack in that dream is simple: plant one tomato. Then another. Then a row of beans, a tub of herbs, and a shelf of jars.

The goal is a personal food safety system, built one bed, one jar, and one habit at a time. You keep going until the store becomes a backup instead of a lifeline, and the next crisis on the news barely dents what you eat.

Chapter 16 Backyard Grass Quick-Start

Turning Lawns Into Food Beds

Some readers reach this point and still see nothing but grass. No beds. No tubs. No old garden corner. Just a strip or square of shaved lawn and a question. Where do you even start? That is a real starting line, and it deserves a direct answer.

A grass yard can move in more than one direction. You can break the sod once and build in the ground. You can skip the tiller and stack a bed on top. You can leave the lawn where it is and grow in large above ground pots, bins, and soft pools while the rest of the yard changes more slowly. Earlier chapters already laid out the pieces. This chapter puts you in a backyard full of grass, wondering where the first cut should go.

The point is not to turn every yard into a perfect grid. The point is to move land away from mowing and toward feeding. Start with one strip, one corner, one pool, or one row of large pots if that is what your time and body allow. A small start still shifts power away from the lawn and back toward the plate.

Some ground is so tight with old sod, roots, and compacted fill that a one time till makes sense. This is not a permission slip for yearly rototilling. It is a short opening move for the grower who wants in ground beds and needs to break the first crust without spending weeks chopping by hand.

Start by mowing the grass as low as possible. Rake heavy clumps, pick up rocks, and pull out junk that can jam blades or wrap around the machine. Mark the beds and walkways before you do anything else. A hose, line of stakes, or dusting of marking paint can save a lot of crooked work later. Once the tiller starts bouncing, people forget where paths were meant to be and chew up more ground than they planned.

Work only when the soil is moist enough to break apart but not so wet that it smears. Watch your step ahead and put on boots if needed. If a handful forms a sticky lump, wait. If it falls through your fingers like ash, wait again, and water first, or wait for rain. Set the tiller to a shallow depth, just deep enough to cut the sod and loosen the upper layer. This is not mining. You are opening the skin, not tearing apart the whole body beneath it.

Make one slow pass, then stop and look. If the sod is broken and the upper layer loosens enough to accept compost and roots, stop there. If a few strips remain too tough, touch only those spots again. Many people make the mistake that this book already warned about. They keep grinding until the whole bed becomes powder. That looks clean for a week, then turns into a crust, a slump, and a loss. One shallow opening is enough.

Right after that pass, spread compost, leaf humus, aged manure, or reused potting mix over the future bed. Rake it into the top few inches and no deeper. From that day forward, the tiller should be finished with that space. The next steps belong to mulch, roots, compost, worms, and time. If you keep coming back with steel every spring, you undo the healing you were trying to start.

Once the bed lines are set, the walkways become their own decision. Some growers want clean paths with less work. Others want living strips that act like soil banks, seed banks, and small nurseries. Either route can work if you understand the trade.

One option is to leave the paths alive. Mow them, trim them, and let them stay soil and roots. Over time, those strips become more than places to step. Clippings feed the surface. Roots loosen the ground. If a few plants are allowed to flower and set seed, the wind helps you. Seeds drift, settle, and wait. In spring, free starts show up in the walkways and along the rough seams where beds meet paths.

That free nursery is not a theory. Volunteer starts appear in rough edges and walkway spaces. Some get lifted with a trowel and moved into pots or better spots before they are crowded out. Earlier chapters already described similar seedlings along torn fabric and container edges, where spilled mix, dried weeds, and stray seed become a nursery if you watch at the right time.

Living paths also give you a simple place to recycle pulled weeds. When weeds come out of the beds, drop them into the walks. Hot sun dries them, kills the roots, and turns them into part of the recycling layer. What looked like a cleanup starts becoming future soil. The cost is maintenance. A living path can help you, but it can also get wild if you stop editing it. Some volunteers belong in pots. Some belong in compost. Some must die before they set seed and become next month's problem.

The cleaner route is to cover the walkways. Lay down filter fabric, cardboard, or another barrier and cover it with wood chips or straw. The path stays neater. Shoes stay cleaner. Less time goes into pulling path weeds. The chips or straw do not just sit there looking tidy. They become a working stockpile for the rest of the yard.

Path cover can be pulled onto exposed bed or pot soil to cut evaporation and block weed light. It can also serve for winter protection. Straw or loose chips can be packed around garlic tubs, laid over winter crops, or banked against containers to soften cold snaps. After a couple of years, the lower chip layer darkens and edges toward the soil. When a walkway gets too rich or too thick, shovel some of it up and put it back to work.

A wood chip walkway can become part of the pot system. When chips start to turn toward soil, move that part in spring while you are already topping off pots, pool beds, and tubs. Put the more broken material into the bottoms of large pots where slow breakdown is welcome, then refresh the walkway with new chips. Containers built on leaf humus and other organic matter sink each year as life consumes the old material. Volume disappears and must be replaced.

In practice, one pot may get dumped into others because the mix has sunk too much to keep that vessel full on its own. Some years, the soil line drops enough that a few empty pots appear. That is when half-composted path material can fill the lower space, save good upper mix for roots, and keep the cycle moving. The walks stay pleasant to use, help with weed control, and later come back as volume and fertility. The path ultimately feeds the pot.

Some growers do not want to break the sod at all. That choice fits this book well because the healing mound idea already showed how to build upward over dead or compacted ground instead of digging deeper and deeper.

Start by mowing the grass low where the bed will go. Then lay down overlapping cardboard or heavy paper over the marked bed area. Do not worry if the surface looks rough. The point is to dim the grass, not to make a showroom floor. On top of that paper skin, build a loose lower layer from rough yard debris. Small sticks, dry stalks, sunflower stems, prunings, and other coarse material work well. They create pockets, hold some air, and begin the slow rot that turns a dead patch into a living mound.

Above that, pile richer material. Compost, leaf humus, aged manure, and used potting mix can all help build the upper rooting layer. Shape it into a low mound or broad bed with enough depth for roots to find footing while the lower layers soften. Finish with surface armor. Straw, chopped leaves, and broken plant residue shield the top, just as earlier chapters argued again and again.

This route requires more patience than a tiller, but it keeps the lower layer of the soil more intact. Old grass dies down. The paper weakens. Roots push through. The bed starts feeding itself. If you have time and enough organic matter, this is often the better long game. It trades machine noise for biology.

Not every reader wants to carve beds into the yard right away. Some want quick production with less digging. Some have rules, hard fill, tree roots, or a body that does not want to fight sod. That is where the large above-ground system comes in.

Small pots look cheap and easy, but they come with their own tax. They dry out fast, overheat, cool quickly, and demand constant watering. A tiny container can turn gardening into a chain around your ankle in the middle of July. Larger vessels behave better. More volume means slower water loss, gentler temperature swings, and more room for roots to find moisture after a hot day.

For that reason, the better route is to go large from the start. Twenty, thirty, fifty, and even one hundred-gallon pots or soft pools make more sense than a crowd of little cans. Earlier chapters already worked at that scale, using 40-gallon tubs, larger pools, and other above-grade systems because they hold steady and can be rebuilt season after season.

Large vessels can also be insulated from the outside. Straw packed around the walls helps retain moisture, soften temperature swings, and give winter roots a better chance when the cold hits hard. Boards, leaves, or other simple outer layers can do a similar job. The goal is not beauty. The goal is to keep the root zone from baking in summer and freezing in winter.

The lower part of a big pot does not have to be filled with the finished mix from the top to the bottom. That space can work for you. While cleaning the yard, rough debris can be recycled into the bottoms of large pots.

Pulled weeds before they seed, soft trimmings, dry stems, small sticks, shredded cardboard, old wood chips, and other light plant waste can all go down low as a rough base. Hay can fill the bottom third when weeds and trimmings run short. The upper rooting layer still needs a real growing mix, but the bottom can become a slow compost zone.

Slow composting turns cleanup waste into future soil. They make the pot lighter than it would be if packed solid with wet earth. Large containers can still be moved with a small dolly when needed. The rough lower layer saves volume at the bottom, where tender roots do not need a fine mix on day one. It also creates a long breakdown zone that feeds the container over time instead of all at once.

The rule is simple. Rougher, lighter material goes low. Better compost and a better mix go higher, where young roots spend the first part of the season. Then the surface gets mulch or cover like any other bed. This is not throwing garbage in a pot and hoping for magic. It is layered by function. The bottom stores carbon and air pockets. The middle starts digestion. The top grows the crop.

A pot built this way changes from year to year. The first season, it is mostly a container with a rough base and a good upper root zone. By the next year, that lower layer begins to settle. The soil line drops a little. That is not failure. That is the system working.

When the level sinks, which it will, especially if you use leaf humus, add more compost, leaf humus, or fresh mix to the top and plant again. Let the lower layers keep breaking down. Each season, the pot becomes less a manufactured container and more a small soil engine.

After two or three years, or whenever the vessel needs it, tip the pot out or dig deep enough to inspect the lower layers. What was once weeds, stems, chips, and scraps has often turned into dark, rich material. That is the moment to flip the system. The old bottom becomes good soil. Part of it can move higher into the root zone or into other beds and pots. Then a new, rough lower-layer GIS is added, and the cycle begins again.

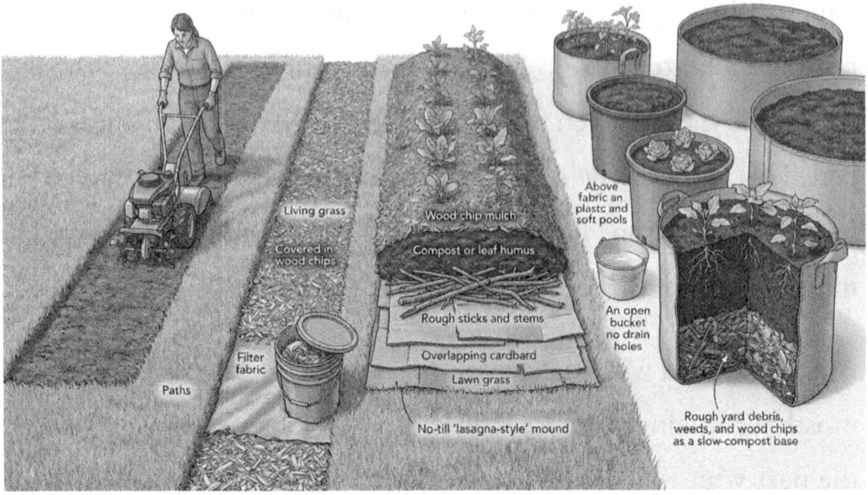

That move turns waste twice. First, it fills volume and keeps the pot lighter. Later, it comes back as real soil. The same path material that once kept shoes clean can end up in the lower layers of a container. The same weeds that once annoyed you can come back as fertility if they were cut before seeding.

Water needs a short word here because a backyard full of grass often becomes a garden in stages, and the first hot spell can catch a beginner off guard. Everyone develops a different rain system. One simple way is to leave containers around the garden with no drain holes so they catch water whenever the sky gives it. That stored water is not fancy, but in an emergency, it is already there. You can grab a bucket and water something without turning on any hoses, sprinklers, or irrigation systems.

Earlier chapters already leaned hard on water capture and drought defense, from drums under gutters to improvised storage and careful triage in dry spells. Small catch pots fit that same logic on a smaller scale. They buy you a fast response. In a sudden dry stretch, a little ready water near the plants beats a perfect plan that exists only on paper.

Kitchen scraps deserve one more place in this chapter because not every yard has room for a full compost setup, and some growers want fertility right where the roots are. A small worm farm or in-place digester can do that work. Earlier chapters described worm rich compost, in bed digesters, half buried buckets with drilled holes, and compost cores that turn scraps into usable fertility near the plants.

A simple version can be made from a large pot, bucket, or cylinder set where you have room in the garden. Layer kitchen scraps with dry leaves, shredded paper, or old straw. Keep meat, grease, and dairy out. Add worms if you have them, and let the whole thing sink over time. The contents shrink, darken, and feed the surrounding area. In a larger bed or pool, a mesh compost heart in the center serves the same job on a bigger scale.

That kind of in place feeding matters because it keeps the kitchen tied to the yard. Scraps do not have to travel to a far corner and wait for perfection. They can become part of the daily cycle. Feed the worms. Feed the digester. Feed the core. Then let roots and microbes do the rest. A backyard food system grows stronger every time another waste stream turns inward instead of leaving.

A yard full of grass does not need one perfect answer. It needs a first move that matches your time, body, budget, and patience. If you want in ground beds fast and the sod is brutal, one shallow till may be enough to open the door.

If you want to protect the lower soil and have enough rough material to build up, a no till bed over grass may be the stronger long play. If your site is poor, rented, ruled by convenience, or just not ready for digging, large above ground pots and pools may carry the first harvest while the rest of the yard evolves.

The wrong move is not choosing pots over beds or living paths over wood chips. The wrong move is staying locked on the lawn because no single option feels perfect.

A productive system can begin with one strip of former grass, one mound, one path lined with chips, one worm pot, one rain-catch tub, or one row of large containers with slow-compost bottoms. Start there. Let the first season teach the second. That is how a food yard begins.

CHAPTER 17 HERBS, TEA, AND YEAR-ROUND EATING

WHAT TO DO WITH YOUR FOOD YARD

The garden is not just about summer and fall harvests. A good yard keeps working in winter, at breakfast, with evening tea, and in small jars on the shelf. Once the lawn starts turning into beds and big pots, the next question is simple. What do you do with all this green power? This chapter walks through how herbs, simple tools, and a few new habits turn a grass yard into a year round food and medicine cabinet.

Some plants do not ask permission. The mint family is one of them. Give mint a big pot, and it will try to own it by the end of the season. That is not a problem. That is a factory. Each year, cut it back hard. Use the clippings to root more pots.

If there are too many, move them into smaller containers and set them out front with a simple price sticker. In many places, you are allowed to sell what you grew in your own yard from a small stand or front corner. The same pattern works with other strong herbs. When they try to take over, turn the extra into plants, not trash.

You do not need to buy every container and pool at full price. There is a steady stream of free and cheap vessels moving through most towns. Tree plantings leave large nursery pots behind. Landscapers often have stacks they are glad to get rid of.

Garbage days and bulk pickup weeks put black tubs and old bins on the curb. Markets and yard sales shed planters as trends change. Pay attention to your normal routes, and a container collection grows without draining your savings. A few new pools or pots each season add up to a serious system after a handful of years.

Pests will test anything you build. Deer nose through beds and tug at leaves. Groundhogs chew stems. Raccoons dig. Cats and other visitors cut paths where they want, not where you planned. Air pests show up, too. Some years whiteflies cloud the leaves. In other years, beetles strip sections bare. Small white butterflies float over brassicas, and their young chew the greens down to lace. There is no one fix. There is a set of tools.

Tall steel posts and wire panels form a first line for big animals. Eight foot posts driven with a pounder and eight or sixteen foot long cattle panels can ring off an upper section of the yard. That does not stop every deer, but it makes the easy path harder. Lower garden edges can hide behind rows of big pots and pools. A tight line of tubs around a bed forces ground animals to slow down and work harder to reach the inner crops.

Traps sometimes join the story. A few cages set in known runs catch more than one kind of visitor. Cats, groundhogs, and raccoons wander in. Laws vary, but many people drive those caught animals far away to woods and fields before letting them out. It is not perfect. It is not pretty. It is one way to reduce pressure without poison. Small sheds or tents can also serve as rodent control posts. Old military tents, simple frames, traps, and repellents can turn a storage corner into a mouse- and rat-checkpoint before tools and stored food suffer further damage.

For insects and small flyers, the tools change. Whiteflies hate moving air. A simple box fan pointed through a tunnel of greens makes landing harder. Beetle bag traps hung on the edge of the property pull some of the load away from tender crops. Butterfly nets let you knock down the worst of the white flutterers near brassica beds. The real backbone, though, comes from mixing plants.

Companion planting works very well in a yard of tubs, pools, and mounds. Do not line up twenty tomatoes in a row and expect no one to notice. Break them into groups. Slide herbs between them. Put strong smelling plants like garlic, chives, oregano, and thyme among the main crops. Spread them out rather than keeping them in one herb corner. Many pests dislike certain scents or become confused when the same crop is not planted in a single long strip. A scattered layout makes it harder for trouble to find a smooth run.

Herbs do more than guard. They carry the garden into every month. Heavy herb planting means you are not just growing flavor, you are growing part of your medicine cabinet and daily fuel. Through the season, cut herbs into blocks. Dry them on racks or screens. Dehydrate them in a simple machine when the air is too damp. Grind dry leaves and stems into powder with a strong blender. Store them in jars away from light and heat. Your yard has now moved from fresh sprigs to a year-round supply.

Frozen herbs and vegetables become another line of storage. If time runs short during peak harvest, it is better to wash and freeze tomatoes or chopped peppers in bags than to let them rot while you dream of a perfect canning weekend.

In winter, those bags turn into soup, broth, and sauce stock. Drop frozen tomatoes into a pot with frozen herbs and other vegetables. Let the slow simmer chase off the cold and stretch last summer's work into the lean months.

Tea becomes more than a box on a shelf. With enough herbs, each night can bring a different mix. There is no rule that tea must be green or come in a bag from a store. Catnip, chamomile, mint of all kinds, lemon balm, thyme, and other leaves can form a base and an accent.

You can ask any smart tool to build blends for sleep, headaches, stress, and other common complaints as long as you tell it which plants you actually have. Most people deal with a handful of regular issues. Custom mixes can be built around those patterns.

Brewing can stay simple. A standard coffee maker with a stainless steel reusable filter works well for both small and large batches. Single-cup machines with metal baskets let you brew one mug at a time without using paper. Larger drip pots can run a blend that fills a thermos or pitcher.

Herbs do not dissolve like sugar, so they pass through a filter easily. Once the hot water runs through them, you have the base. Citrus and honey can be added later. Homegrown stevia leaves can sweeten filters or pots, too. They do not melt like crystals but lend sweetness when water passes through or steeps with them.

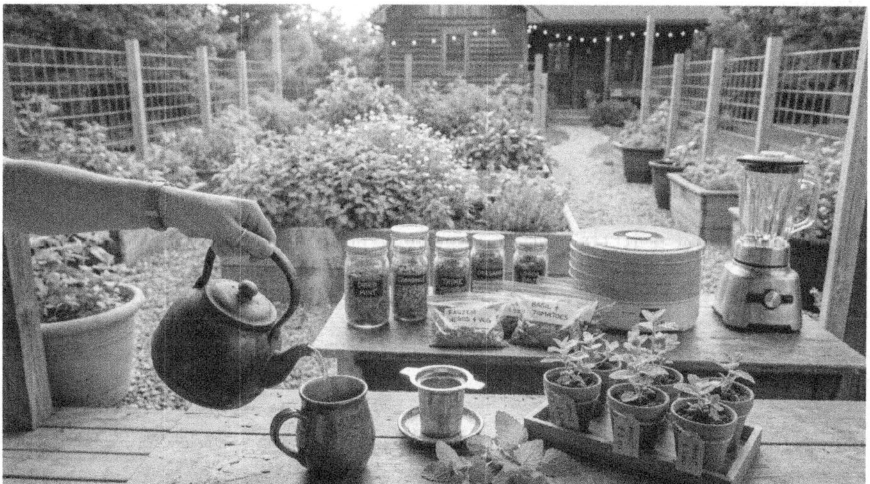

Cooking habits change in the same way. Eggs stop being a blank canvas for only salt and pepper. They receive blends of powdered chives, garlic, parsley, basil, or whatever else fits the meal. Soups, stews, and sauces pick up mixes pulled from jars you filled yourself. Breadings, rubs, and even simple sandwiches step into another world once you shake on herb blends that grew ten yards from the table.

The plate fills with more color and more real plant matter without a single extra pill.

When a yard works this way, bags and bottles from stores lose some of their grip. Many commercial teas and spices contain preservatives, dyes, pesticides, and fillers that are never needed. Some blends even use sand or other grip agents to keep them flowing in machines. Vegetables in stores often arrive waxed, coated, tired, and carrying a history you will never read on the label. This is not about never buying another carrot. It is about cutting that dependency and thinking more carefully about what you bring home.

Other books lay out, in more detail, how store-bought food and restaurant dishes can carry hidden loads that harm over time. The point here is shorter. Every spoonful and sip from your own yard cuts that load a little more. Every jar of dried thyme, every bag of frozen tomatoes, every cup of mixed tea is a small move away from a system that treats you like a unit on a balance sheet.

This path also pushes on how you spend money and time. You do not need a full set of machines and tools in year one. A strong blender, a simple dehydrator, a secondhand freezer, a basic vacuum sealer, or even a freeze dryer, if luck and funds allow, can arrive over several seasons. Most of these show up in used condition at estate sales, online markets, pawn shops, or garage sales. Pots and tools come the same way. Slow collection beats big debt.

Time shifts with it. The hours you once spent on glowing screens and store aisles can be spent outside. Turning off the television, cutting back on social media time, and skipping trips to buy things you do not truly need create space. A food yard does ask for work, but much of it can replace work that never fed you in the first place. Spending less on empty things means you can afford to work less or at least feel less cornered by your bills.

Real rest looks different, too. Vacation ads show beaches, drinks, and sand from other countries. There is nothing wrong with a break, but that glitter often fades fast. A chair in your own garden, watching bees move through flowers you planted, smelling herbs in the evening air, and knowing jars and bags in the kitchen came from your hands, carries a different weight. It does not vanish when the plane lands. It sits in the soil, season after season.

None of these demands perfection. You will lose crops to pests. Deer will jump a fence. Whiteflies will win some rounds. Some tea mixes will taste strange. A batch of dried herbs may mold if you rush the process. The freezer may ice over. You may miss a week of the wedding when life goes sideways. That does not erase the gains. A yard that used to feed only a mower can now feed a year's mind, and a year's worth of meals and cups. Every small step away from the lawn and toward food counts.

A Note from the Author

If this book helped you grow more food, think differently about your soil, or feel a little less trapped by the grocery aisles, I would be grateful if you left a brief positive review on Amazon. Reviews are not just about ego. They are the only real way many readers ever find books like this in a crowded search page.

Most people who enjoy a book never leave a single sentence behind, and the algorithms quietly bury quiet voices. A few honest lines, from you, in your own words, can help other families discover these ideas, start their own small systems, and rely a little less on the same fragile chains you are trying to escape.

If you have suggestions, questions, or ideas for future topics, you are welcome to mention those as well. Your feedback shapes what I write next and helps me keep these books practical, blunt, and worth your time.

Further Reading by Marko Vovk

This book is part of a larger project to help ordinary people take back control of their homes, health, and food. If you found it useful, you may also like these titles. To find any of them, search for **"Marko Vovk"** on Amazon.

Current Books

Above-Ground Gardening – Growing Food Without Digging Up Your Yard (2026)
A practical guide to tubs, pools, and containers that turn dead corners into productive food systems without tilling up your yard.

Pressure Canning – Safe Preservation of Food at Home (2026)
A step by step handbook on canning low acid foods and full meals safely, with clear explanations of gear, tested recipes, and risk points.

Poisoned at the Grocery Store – Why Shopping Fresh Is Not Enough to Escape a Toxic Food Supply (2025)
Explores how chemicals, processing, coatings, and packaging follow

you even into the "healthy" aisles, and what it takes to build a safer food pipeline.

No-Mow Living – The Real Hidden Costs of Grass (2025)
Looks at how lawns waste water, fuel, and time, and shows how to convert turf into beds, paths, and low care spaces that actually serve your life.

The Water You Drink May Be Killing You (2024)
Examines contaminants in tap and bottled water, how they reach your glass, and what you can do at the house level to reduce exposure.

The Water You Drink May Be Killing You (2023)
Explores how industrial discharges, old pipes, and regulatory gaps can turn safe looking water into a chronic burden on your body.

Forever Chemicals – How PFAS Pollutes Our Blood and Lives (2023)
Unpacks how PFAS moves from factories into food, water, and homes, and why it is so hard to escape once it is in the environment.

Surviving Electrosmog – How to Understand and Reduce Invisible Pollution in Your Home and Life (2024)
Explains everyday exposures from wireless and electrical systems, and offers practical steps to reduce them without moving off grid.

Fix Your Toxic Home and Live Longer (2022)
Walks through pollutants hidden in building materials, finishes, and furnishings, and how to make a normal house safer over time.

Make Your Home Great Again (For Homeowners and Buyers) – Expanded Tips Edition (2023)

Collects decades of inspection experience into checklists and advice for finding, fixing, and maintaining homes that do not quietly harm you.

Don't Rent This Home, Condo, or Apartment (2023)

A renter focused guide to spotting structural, moisture, and environmental red flags before you sign a lease.

Bias: How Our Minds Deceive Us – 18 Ways Your Perceptions Are Skewed and How to See More Clearly (2024)

Shows how cognitive biases shape what we notice, what we ignore, and how we make decisions about risk, money, and health.

Childless Cat Lady – Movement, Dynamics, Health, and Political Influence (2024)

Looks at demographic change, shifting family patterns, and how online culture around pets and childlessness spills into politics.

Nuclear Extinction Event Is Killing Our Families' Pets: The Hidden Costs of Companionship (2024)

Examines how indoor pet culture intersects with toxins, stress, and health costs for both animals and the people who love them.

Project 2025 Quick Review (2024)

A fast, plain language walkthrough of Project 2025 themes and what they could mean for ordinary households and rights.

Empty Cradles – Declining Birth Rates Explained (2026)
Connects medical, environmental, economic, and cultural forces that converge into falling birth rates and aging societies.

The Duck Who Watched (2026)
A reality fiction novel about a porch duck that quietly watches the houses across the street, using one bird's vantage point to explore family, secrets, and neighborhood change.

The Sixth Extinction: Return to Earth 2225 (2025)
Dystopian fiction about how the Anunnaki return to a scarred Earth with only 500,000 people left, tying modern environmental damage to a future where an old presence comes back to a nearly emptied planet.

Moon Sense – How Lunar Cycles Nudge Sleep, Mood, and Daily Life (2026)
A plain language look at how moon phases may line up with small shifts in how people sleep, feel, and plan, written for curious but skeptical readers.

White Papers

Hidden Drivers of Population Decline – How Modern Health, Environmental, and Medical Risks Create Empty Cradles (2026)
Connects toxins, chronic illness, and subtle reproductive harms into one picture of falling birth rates.

Indoor Pets, Hidden Costs – Health, Housing, Money, and the Environment in Pet-Centric Living (2026)
Looks at the unseen financial, health, and environmental impacts of modern pet culture.

Earth Helpers Kids' Series (from 2025)

Short, direct books that help kids see hidden risks and helpers in the modern world:

EMF KIDS – The Secret World of Invisible Waves

Grass KIDS – Why the Lawn Isn't Always Greener

Home Safety KIDS – Smart Habits for Everyday Dangers

Lucky to Be Alive – Discover Why Every Life Is a Miracle

Nuclear KIDS – Little Lessons from Atomic Power

PFAS KIDS – The Forever Chemical Mystery

The Great Smoke, Fire & Dust Adventure

The Vitamin ABC's – A Healthy Kids' Guide

Eight additional Earth Helpers Kids' Series titles are planned for 2026–2027.

Glossary

Amendment
Any material you add to soil or potting mix to improve structure, drainage, or fertility, such as compost, leaf mold, or aged manure.

Anhydrous ammonia
A concentrated nitrogen fertilizer gas injected into soil, originally produced for explosives and later sold as "plant food."

Armor (soil armor)
Any protective cover on the soil surface—mulch, crop residue, or living plants—that shields ground from sun, wind, and pounding rain.

Biochar
Charcoal made from plant material and added to soil to hold nutrients and water and give microbes extra habitat.

Canning (water bath)
Preserving high acid foods like pickles, jams, jellies, and many tomato products in jars processed in boiling water to make them shelf stable.

Canning (pressure)
Preserving low acid foods such as vegetables, meats, and full meals in jars processed under pressure so they reach higher, botulism-killing temperatures.

Chop and drop
A method where you cut spent plants and weeds, leave the roots in place, and drop the tops on the surface as mulch instead of hauling them away.

Compost
Decomposed plant material made from layered "greens" and "browns" that turns into dark, crumbly matter used to feed soil and improve structure.

Compost core
A tube or pocket of raw organic scraps buried inside a bed or container so that the garden "eats" kitchen waste from the inside out.

Cover crop
A crop planted mainly to protect and feed soil instead of to harvest, often used to add organic matter, fix nitrogen, prevent erosion, and smother weeds.

Dead zone
An area in a lake or ocean where fertilizer-driven algae blooms use up oxygen so severely that most aquatic life cannot survive.

Exudates
Sugars and other compounds that plant roots leak into the surrounding soil to feed microbes in exchange for nutrients and protection.

Fertilizer (synthetic)
Industrial salts made in factories and sold as quick "plant food," usually supplying nitrogen, phosphorus, and potassium in bagged form.

Forest inoculation
The practice of sprinkling a small amount of healthy forest soil onto damaged ground or beds to introduce diverse microbes and fungi.

Heirloom seed
Open pollinated seed from older varieties that reliably grow "true to type" and can be saved and replanted year after year.

Hybrid seed
Seed produced by crossing two inbred parent lines for one generation of strong performance; saved seed usually splits and does not stay true.

Keyhole garden
A round raised bed with a notch ("keyhole") for access and a compost

basket at the center that turns kitchen scraps and rinse water into steady fertility.

Lasagna bed / mound
A no till bed built by stacking layers of rough organic matter and richer materials on top of existing ground, like a pan of lasagna.

Legume
Plants such as beans, peas, and clover that host nitrogen fixing bacteria on their roots and can add nitrogen to soil.

Leaching
The loss of nutrients as water carries them down and out of the root zone, often from bare or over-fertilized soil.

Mulch
Any material laid on top of soil—straw, leaves, wood chips, chopped plants—to conserve moisture, suppress weeds, and protect the surface.

Mycorrhizae
Fungi that form partnerships with plant roots and send out fine threads to collect water and nutrients in exchange for sugars.

Nitrogen fixation
The process by which certain bacteria associated with legumes turn nitrogen from the air into forms plants can use in the soil.

Open pollinated
Varieties in which plants of the same type pollinate naturally so saved

urally so saved seed grows plants similar to the parents, as long as you avoid crossing with other types.

Rhizosphere
The thin zone of soil right around plant roots where exudates, microbes, and nutrient trading are most concentrated.

Rotational pots / above-grade gardens
A system where you grow crops in containers, pools, or tubs above ground and rotate what grows in them instead of tilling fixed in--ground rows.

Seed bank (home)
Your personal stash of saved and purchased seeds kept cool, dark, and dry so you can replant future gardens even if store racks are empty.

Soil food web
The entire underground community of microbes, fungi, insects, worms, and other creatures that recycle organic matter and feed plants.

Tilth
The feel and workability of soil—how crumbly, loose, and well-structured it is when you dig or plant into it.

Trap crop
A plant you deliberately grow to attract pests away from main crops so you can monitor and remove infestations in a controlled spot.

Three Sisters

An Indigenous planting system that grows corn, climbing beans, and squash together so they share light, roots, nutrients, and protection.

Topdressing

A thin layer of compost or other amendment spread on top of soil around plants to feed and improve the surface without digging.

Bibligraphy

Berry, Wendell. *The Unsettling of America: Culture and Agriculture*. San Francisco, CA: Sierra Club Books, 1977.

Briggs, Dan. "Fireplace Ashes on Your Soil." Baton Rouge, LA: LSU AgCenter, 2005.

Brown, Gabe. *Dirt to Soil: One Family's Journey into Regenerative Agriculture*. White River Junction, VT: Chelsea Green Publishing, 2018.

Chalker-Scott, Linda. "Compost Tea: Miracle or Myth?" Seattle, WA: Washington State University Extension, ca. 2007.

Consortium for Southern Africa Food Security Emergency (C-SAFE) and CARE. *Keyhole Gardens in Lesotho and Zimbabwe: Project Reports and Field Guides*. 2006–2013.

Diaz, Robert J., and Rutger Rosenberg. "Spreading Dead Zones and Consequences for Marine Ecosystems." *Science* 321, no. 5891 (2008): 926–929.

Earlham Institute. Seaton, D. D., et al. "Geographical Patterns of DNA Methylation in Global Wheat Collections." Norwich, UK: Earlham Institute, 2018.

ECHO. "Keyhole Garden." ECHOcommunity technical note. 2008.

Evergreen Seniors. "The $0 Garden That Killed Raised Beds — Why Every Garden Store Hides This Method." YouTube video, 26:49, accessed 2026.

Fan, Dongdong, et al. "Effects of Seaweed Fertilizers on Crop Yield and Quality: A Meta-Analysis." *Agronomy* (or similar; insert final journal details when confirmed), 2024.

Fukuoka, Masanobu. *The One Straw Revolution: An Introduction to Natural Farming*. Emmaus, PA: Rodale Press, 1978.

Green America. "What Practices Make My Garden a Climate Victory Garden?" Washington, DC: Green America, 2025.

Grossman, Elizabeth. "Gee Whiz: Human Urine Is Shown to Be an Effective Agricultural Fertilizer." *Scientific American*, July 23, 2010.

Hoitink, Harry A. J., and A. G. Stone. "Use of Compost and Compost Teas for Plant Disease Suppression." Wooster, OH: Ohio State University / OARDC, 2000.

Howard, Sir Albert. *An Agricultural Testament*. New York, NY: Oxford University Press, 1943.

Jeavons, John. *How to Grow More Vegetables*. 9th ed. Berkeley, CA: Ten Speed Press, 2017.

Khan, Wajid, Upendra P. Rayirath, Subramanian Subramanian, et al. "Seaweed Extracts as Biostimulants of Plant Growth and Development." *Journal of Applied Phycology* 21, no. 5 (2009): 561–573.

Kimbrell, Andrew, ed. *Fatal Harvest: The Tragedy of Industrial Agriculture*. Washington, DC: Island Press, 2002.

Lapham's Quarterly. "Leftovers." *Lapham's Quarterly*, Winter 2004.

Larsen, Thomas A., et al. "Fertilizers from Recycled Human Urine Are Safe and Effective for Cabbage Cultivation." *Frontiers in Environmental Science* 11 (2023).

Mary Robinson Foundation – Climate Justice. "How a 'Joined-up' Approach, Centred on Keyhole Gardens, Is Tackling Hunger and Climate Change in Lesotho." Briefing paper, 2013.

Master Gardeners of Northern Virginia. "Cover Crops to Enrich Soil." Arlington, VA: MGNV, 2023.

Michigan State University Extension. "Understanding Companion, Trap and Cover Crops: A Guide for Home Gardeners." East Lansing, MI: MSU Extension, 2026.

Mohler, Charles L., and Kimberly A. Stoner. *The Three Sisters Mound System* (sometimes cited as "The Science Behind the Three

Sisters Mound System"). Ithaca, NY: Cornell-linked research PDF, ca. 2015–2018.

Mt. Pleasant, Jane. "The Three Sisters Cropping System: An Indigenous Agricultural Practice." Lecture and associated materials. Ithaca, NY: Cornell University, ca. 2015.

National Garden Bureau. "Victory Garden 2.0: Soil Basics." Downers Grove, IL: National Garden Bureau, 2025.

Netherlands Institute of Ecology (NIOO-KNAW). "Soil Organisms Steer Ecosystem Restoration." Wageningen, Netherlands: NIOO press release summarizing Wubs et al. 2016.

Penn State Extension. "Tips for Planting Cover Crops in Home Gardens." University Park, PA: Penn State Extension, 2026.

Phelps, Leonard. "Wood Ashes for the Home Garden." Burlington, VT: University of Vermont Extension, 2023.

Pollan, Michael. *The Omnivore's Dilemma: A Natural History of Four Meals.* New York, NY: Penguin Press, 2006.

Pradhan, Surendra K., and Helvi Heinonen-Tanski. "Human Urine and Wood Ash as Plant Nutrients for Red Beet (Beta vulgaris)." *Journal of Agricultural and Food Chemistry* 58, no. 3 (2010): 865–871.

Reeves, Walter. "Compost Tea – Does It Work?" *The Georgia Gardener,* June 19, 2020.

Rodale Institute and Pennsylvania State University. "Evaluation of Compost Tea for Crop Growth and Disease Suppression." Kutztown, PA: Rodale Institute, ca. 2000–2005.

Rosen, Carl J., and Mark E. Stolt. "Guide to Using Wood Ash as an Agricultural Soil Amendment." Durham, NH: University of New Hampshire Extension, 2025.

Salatin, Joel. *You Can Farm: The Entrepreneur's Guide to Start and Succeed in a Farming Enterprise*. Swoope, VA: Polyface Inc., 1998.

Seaton, D. D., et al. See Earlham Institute entry above (epigenetics in wheat collections).

Send a Cow Lesotho. *Keyhole Gardens in Lesotho for Better Nutrition and Food Security*. Project fact sheet, 2010.

Stone Pier Press. "The Might of Tiny Victory Gardens." San Francisco, CA: Stone Pier Press, 2021.

Tennessee Valley Authority / University of North Alabama Archives. *Tennessee Valley Authority: A Technological History of United States Nitrate Plant No. 2*. Muscle Shoals, AL: TVA/UNA Archives, ca. 2013.

"TVA: The Great Experiment." PDH Online, technical course C797, ca. 2010.

United Nations Convention to Combat Desertification. *Global Land Outlook*. Bonn, Germany: UNCCD, 2017.

United States Department of Agriculture. *The 1943 Victory Garden Program*. Washington, DC: U.S. Government Printing Office, 1943.

United States Department of Agriculture. *Victory Gardens*. Washington, DC: U.S. Government Printing Office, 1943.

United States Department of Agriculture, Agricultural Research Service. "Time for Victory Gardens Again?" *Scientific Discoveries*, 2019.

United States Department of Agriculture, National Agricultural Library. "Victory Gardens and Farms." Special Collections exhibit. Beltsville, MD: NAL, 2020.

United States Department of Agriculture. "Victory Gardens: Food for the Fight." The National WWII Museum online article, 2024.

United States Environmental Protection Agency. "Nutrient Pollution: The Gulf of Mexico Dead Zone." Technical report, latest revision.

United States Federal Public Housing Authority. *Victory Gardens for Tenants of Housing Projects*. Washington, DC: FPHA, 1943.

University of Georgia Extension. "Winter Cover Crops in Raised Garden Beds." Athens, GA: UGA Extension, 2025.

University of Maine Cooperative Extension. "Victory Garden for ME." Orono, ME: UMaine Extension, 2020–2024 series.

University of New Hampshire Extension. "Fertilizing Vegetable Gardens." Durham, NH: UNH Extension, 2025.

Vovk, Marko. *Grass Be Gone*. Self-published, Amazon KDP, year of publication.

Vovk, Marko. *No Mow Living*. Self-published, Amazon KDP, year of publication.

Vovk, Marko. *Poisoned at the Grocery Store: What They Added and Never Told You*. Self-published, Amazon KDP, year of publication.

Vovk, Marko. *Poisoned at the Restaurant* (if published; remove this line if not yet in print). Self-published, Amazon KDP, year of publication.

Vovk, Marko. *[Final Title of This Book]*. Self-published, Amazon KDP, 2026.

Wubs, E. R. J., W. H. van der Putten, M. Bosch, and T. M. Bezemer. "Soil Inoculation Steers Restoration of Terrestrial Ecosystems." *Nature Plants* 2 (2016): 16107.

Made in the USA
Monee, IL
04 November 2026

67386619R00075